# The Fine Print of Fibro

Amanda Leanne

Published by Mune's Quill, 2017.

THE FINE PRINT OF FIBRO

**First edition. October 15, 2017.**



ISBN: 979-8215497692

Written by Amanda Leanne.

# Table of Contents

As this is my first official published book, under my own name and not a ghostwriter job, I was a bit nervous about making a dedication. There are a lot of people that have helped me and there are even more that hurt me. A few people, though, really made me push through it all to get this far. The first is my son, Adeon. Without him, I would have given up so long ago. Secondly, but not less by any means, is my partner Kris. He has been more than supportive of me dedicating myself to my writing and has always stood by me with everything I have been through since I met him. I look forward to many years with this man, and many more dedications mentioning him. I also have to thank my father, who passed away a few years ago, and my mom, for nurturing my thirst to read and write since I was a child, and for that first typewriter I got for Christmas so many years ago. There are many others, but I didn't want to go on and on. So to my family and friends I haven't mentioned, I appreciate what all of you have done for me, good or bad, as it made me who I am today.

Thank you all so much.

Special side note to another Fibromyalgia warrior who just suffered the devastating sudden loss of her partner in life and the father of her children, Dee. She is more than a warrior and her battles have only gotten harder. Much love and good wishes to her and her family.

# Table of Contents

## Preface

There are already a ton of websites, books, eBooks, and other materials out there on Fibromyalgia. So why did I write mine? Honestly, I felt like people needed something a bit more "real" to read. I am blunt by nature, forward thinking and not a big sugar-coater. I have explained this disease to many people of all ages. Some were diagnosed and never explained what they have and what that meant. I have had people list of all kinds of issues and follow every one with the question "is that fibro related?"

With that being said, I decided to combine my knowledge and experience into a book to help people that are unsure of what to expect, what it is, and how other people learn to cope with having Fibromyalgia.

I have a disclaimer on the copyright page but I want to remind my readers that I am not a doctor or medical professional. I do have certifications in first responder, phlebotomy, and some other random areas, but I am not a professional. Serious medical issues and problems need to be brought to the attention of your doctor. If it is an emergency, please call your emergency number or go to the emergency room. I am not to blame for ill taken advice or the use of my words when it comes to your health.

Thank you all so much!

# THE FINE PRINT OF FIBRO

Some words are in *italics*. The definitions and/or explanations of these words are listed below. Some of the words still have a brief explanation after them, but this section gives a bit more information and detail. I hope this helps with any confusion with some of the slang and medical words that are found in this book.

<u>Anemia</u> – Health condition where blood is lacking healthy red blood cells

<u>CBD (cannabidiol)</u> – CBD is a chemical found in marijuana that is much less psychoactive than THC. CBD is used medically to help with anxiety, depression, pain, muscle spasms, headaches, migraines, insomnia, nausea, and even epilepsy. Indicas have a much higher CBD content than THC

<u>Carpal Tunnel Syndrome</u> – Painful condition in which the joints and tendons in your wrist becomes swollen or aggravated from over use or repetitive use.

<u>Catheter</u> – A small tube inserted in the urethra and reaching the bladder to release urine.

<u>Celiac Disease</u> – An autoimmune disease activated by the presence of gluten causing the villi of the intestines to smooth out, damage to the stomach, allergic like reactions to the skin (such as lesions and boils), mood swings, headaches, diarrhea, constipation, urinary issues, swelling and bloating, weight gain, malnutrition (as the body is no longer able to absorb nutrition from ingested foods and fluids).

<u>Cerebral Hematoma</u> – blood pooling in the brain, like a bruise under the skull.

<u>Chrohn's Disease</u> – is a lifelong incurable condition in which the lining of a person's intestines and stomach are easily or always inflamed causing diarrhea, pain, anemia, loss of weight, and many other health issues.

<u>Chronic</u> – Continuing, long term, repeatedly occurring

<u>CFS (chronic fatigue syndrome)</u> – is a health condition similar to Fibro but a bigger emphasis on the fatigue. The person can be perpetually tired and exhausted to the point of pain and any exertion only makes it worse.

<u>Cognitive</u> – mental processes, the actions the mind makes when you read, write, think, talk, use your memory, etc.

<u>Costochondritis</u> – Sharp pains in the chest/sternum area of the body. This is believed to be caused by swelling and aggravation of the cartilage that connects the ribs and breast bone and is also referred to as Tietze Syndrome.

<u>De Quervain's tenosynovitis</u> – is a painful condition in which the tendons that run from your thumb, down through your wrist and arm become swollen or inflamed from use.

<u>Degenerative disc disease</u> – is an incurable disease in which the discs in a person's spine break down, fall apart, or become brittle over time. Causes a lot of pain and can lead to paralysis.

<u>Dopamine</u> – A neurotransmitter that is considered the brain's reward system. When released, it causes pleasant feelings for the person. (This is often released during drug/caffeine/nicotine use, exercise, sex, etc.)

<u>Fibromite</u> – A nickname some people with Fibromyalgia use to refer to themselves.

<u>Fibromyalgia</u> – A musculoskeletal and neurological condition causing pain and fatigue as well as memory, mood, and other health conditions.

<u>Fibro Flare</u> – A time period lasting from hours to weeks in which a person with Fibromyalgia feels extreme levels of pain, sensory issues, sleeplessness, and general overreaction of the nervous system.

<u>Fibro Fog</u> – A time period lasting from hours to weeks in which a person with Fibromyalgia has extreme difficulty with thinking, cognitive skills, memory, concentration, alertness, etc.

<u>Gastrointestinal</u> – The body system involving the stomach, intestines, bowel, etc.

<u>Homeopathic</u> – A "natural" or homemade remedy made from herbs, produce, plants, oils, etc. that is often used in place or to supplement medication.

<u>Hypochondriac</u> – A person who psychologically believes they have physical ailments due to an overactive mental awareness of plausible health issues.

<u>Indica</u> – Strain of marijuana plant with a higher CBD than THC level, often used for medical purposes.

<u>ICS (interstitial cystitis)</u> – is a condition in which the bladder becomes aggravated and inflamed due to almost anything digested by the body. It can cause many symptoms such as frequent urination, painful urination, inability to urinate, difficulty emptying the bladder, abdominal bloating, and even pain with sexual intercourse. The only way to have absolutely no flares of the bladder is a diet consisting of rice, water, and blueberries....a rather ridiculous scenario.

<u>Invisible Illness</u> – An illness, disease, disorder, or condition that cannot be seen by the outside person. Examples are diabetes, cancer, Fibromyalgia, Lupus, Lyme, MS, IBS, ICS, CFS, Chrohn's Disease, etc.

<u>IBS (Irritable Bowel Syndrome)</u> – Can be diarrhea or constipation that occurs for no specific reason or relating to another health condition or medication. IBS is known to act up in stressful situations that are mental, physical or both.

<u>Lupus</u> – A painful and exhausting autoimmune disease in which the body attacks itself. It is incurable. This can sometimes be shown as a red "butterfly" rash that can appear on the face of people that have Lupus. Blood tests do exist for confirmation, though they are not always conclusive. Like CFS, it is often mistaken as Fibromyalgia or vice versa.

<u>Lyme</u> – Bacteria infection caused by a tick bite, usually resulting in a "target" shaped rash where the bite occurs. This results in conditions causing constant pain and illness. Can be treated with antibiotics, but on some occasions the pain issues may remain.

<u>MAO inhibitor</u> – Monoamine oxidase inhibitors are chemicals in medication that is used to treat depression.

MS (multiple sclerosis) – is a disease that takes over the body and causes the immune system to slowly eat away the protective coatings and layers on nerves. The condition is incurable and can cause excruciating pain, constant fatigue, paralysis, breakdown of neurological function. The symptoms can come and go or be permanently active.

Musculoskeletal – Involving both muscles and bones.

Neurotransmitter – A type of chemical in the body that is used to send messages to the brain in order to cause a specific reaction.

NSAID (nonsteroidal anti-inflammatory drug) – these are medications that reduce pain and lower fevers.

Norepinephrine – neurotransmitter that causes fight or flight responses, blood pressure increase, adrenaline release, etc.

Osteomyelitis diskitis – is an infection in the bone and discs of the spine.

OTC (over the counter) – these are medications purchased without a prescription.

Pelvic Prolapse – The disconnection of organs in the pelvis, causing them to drop or fall into the lower areas of the pelvis and sometimes even protrude out of the anus and even the vaginal opening.

Penicillin – A commonly used, strong antibiotic. This has a similar composition to Amoxicillin, and so the allergy to one means an allergy to the other.

Peripheral neuropathy – is pain and weakness in hands and feet due to nerve damage or decay.

PICC Line – is an intravenous ("in the vein"/IV) line that is used to take medication directly to your heart. Similar to "ports" some patients have on their chest for chemotherapy.

Plantar fasciitis – pain in the bottom of the feet, often referred to as the feeling of walking on razor blades (even if your feet are not touching anything).

<u>PCM (primary care manager)</u> – this is the doctor, nurse, or medical professional that is seen on a regular basis, for checkups, for referrals, or any non-specialized visits.

<u>Preeclampsia</u> – A high blood pressure issue with pregnant women that can be fatal to both the mother and the baby.

<u>Psychological</u> – Having to do with a mental reaction and not a physical reaction.

<u>Restless Leg Syndrome</u> – is a neurological condition causing the constant movement or bouncing of the leg.

<u>Rheumatoid Arthritis</u> – Inflammation and pain from swollen joints, usually in the hands and feet.

<u>Sativa</u> – Strain of marijuana often used for recreational purposes and contains a higher amount of THC than CBD.

<u>SSRI (selective serotonin reuptake inhibitor)</u> – Usually found in antidepressants and effects the serotonin release in your brain.

<u>Serotonin</u> – neurotransmitter that deals with sleep, appetite, sex drive, memory, mood, temperature regulation, and behavior.

<u>SIDS (sudden infant death syndrome)</u> – An outdated term used to refer to a death of unknown cause in infants.

<u>Spoonie</u> – A nickname people with Chronic Pain use in reference to the "Spoon Theory" (check the websites section for the information on how to read this neat little story that can help someone with Fibromyalgia, CFS, Lupus, etc. explain to someone, who does not understand, what it is like to have constant fatigue and physical limitations).

<u>Strep B Positive</u> – A bacteria that can be commonly found in the human body but can be fatal to newborns if the mother tests positive. This does not have any effect on the adult carrier.

<u>TMJ (temporomandibular joint disorders)</u> –is a pain in the jaw and lower facial muscles, worse with chewing and talking.

<u>THC (tetrahydrocannabinol)</u> – This is the stimulating chemical in marijuana. THC is credited with causing deeper though, higher

imagination, focus, concentration, and even mental energy. Sativas have a much higher level of THC than CBD.

Vertigo – an imbalance caused by an internal issue in the ear, causes the mind to feel unstable, tilted, or like it is falling even when on level ground. This sometimes can cause visual disturbances of tilting.

# What is Fibromyalgia?

*Fibromyalgia* is considered a *musculoskeletal* and neurological disorder. Several major medical institutions are focusing on the study and understanding of what exactly Fibromyalgia is, how it can be best treated, what causes it, and if there is a possibility of a cure. Currently there is no cure. The methods to diagnose and treat are not an exact science and have ample room for error. There are also other medical conditions that can be misdiagnosed as Fibromyalgia as well as misdiagnosis of other medical conditions that can actually be Fibromyalgia.

Fibro (a shortened reference to Fibromyalgia) sucks. It is not fun, it is difficult to deal with, and much about the disease does face controversy. I will be rather blunt in my writings. This isn't a spiritual book, a dry medical read, or a bunch of ramblings (though I cannot promise that I won't occasionally ramble). This first chapter is about the medical and scientific information about the disease. Some of the information is not considered completely definitive, depending on what country you live in, as some have progressed further than others on the research.

What is really interesting about the medical advances in the area of Fibromyalgia is the fact that less than 25 years ago, it was considered a psychological condition related to being a hypochondriac and was not considered a physical health condition. Luckily we have mostly surpassed this belief and are finally moving forward with having better understanding and medical research on Fibromyalgia. This doesn't mean there aren't still people who do not understand or are willing to believe the condition is a legitimate medical concern. I have met people and professionals in the past few years that still refuse to acknowledge Fibromyalgia. This can be disheartening and difficult to deal with, but we will cover that issue further in the book.

## <u>Medical Definition</u>

The Mayo Clinic defines Fibromyalgia as "a disorder characterized by widespread musculoskeletal pain accompanied by fatigue, sleep, memory and mood issues." *Fibro* is a Latin term used for fibrous tissue, *myo* is the Greek base word for muscle, and *algia* is the Greek base word for pain. The primary terminology used to describe the type of medical issue that Fibromyalgia is labeled as is a *musculoskeletal* disorder.

Fibromyalgia is an issue with the central nervous system, the brain and the spinal nerves. Fibro patients have a surplus of an overactive *neurotransmitter* referred to as substance P. This neurotransmitter is found in the spinal fluid and is part of the transmission and processing of the signals relating to pain being taken to and from the brain. With the excess of substance P, there is an excess of pain reactions by the body. Fibro patients also tend to have low *serotonin* (behavior, wants, needs, etc.) and *dopamine* (the "reward" chemical) neurotransmitter levels but excessive *norepinephrine* (fight or flight, anxiety, blood pressure regulation) neurotransmitter levels. These all cause a higher sensitivity to pain and overreaction to pain and any other neurological stimulations and senses.

The way I describe Fibromyalgia to people is to picture the nervous system as electrical wiring through your body. Picture the brain as a fuse box. With Fibro, the wires have spots where the protective rubber or plastic is missing and the wire is exposed, maybe even frayed. What happens is that occasionally these wires touch or an arch of electricity jumps from one wire to another. This causes lights or outlets that the wires go to flicker or buzz, and in some cases, even trip the breaker in the box. So when the wires touch or arch, our nervous system is sparking. This is why we feel random pain or worse pain than normal. This also results in other sensations like temperature issues (being too hot or too cold or unable to handle one or both easily), skin sensations that feel like tickling or spider webs, burning sensations, numbness and tingling, spasms, and so on. A flare or fog would be the instances where the breaker is "flipped" or the fuse blows. This same analogy can be used to refer to the psychological aspects of Fibromyalgia. Chemicals in the brain are pumped at levels that are unnaturally high or unnaturally low. This combined with the pain and overactive nerve sensations (especially since there is no visible rash, bruise or sign to explain the feelings) can cause anxiety and depression. Outside factors like dependency on medication, inability to do things you used to do or want to do, and how people react towards you can also influence the psychological aspects of Fibromyalgia, which in turn can make the physical symptoms worse and on and on in an endless cycle.

## <u>Common Symptoms</u>

- Fatigue
- Waking up tired/unrested
- Insomnia
- Difficulty sleeping and staying asleep because of pain
- Migraines
- Tension headaches
- TMJ (*temporomandibular joint disorders*)
- IBS (*irritable bowel syndrome*) (chronic constipation and/or diarrhea)
- Anxiety
- Depression
- Widespread pain
- *Cognitive* difficulties and dysfunction
- Abdominal pain and cramping
- Joint pain and stiffness (especially upon waking or after being immobile for a bit)
- Muscle pain
- Low pain threshold
- Sensory sensitivity (light, sounds, smell, touch, taste)
- Temperature sensitivity and difficulty regulating (freezing,

overheating, etc.)

- Muscle spasms
- *Costochondritis* (chest pain and sensitivity)
- Memory problems
- Numbness and tingling in hands and feet, or other parts of the body
- *Restless leg syndrome*
- Skin sensitive to touch (itchy, burning, and/or pain)
- Concentration issues
- *ICS* (interstitial cystitis) or bladder pain and/or frequency
- Reduced exercise due to pain or fatigue it causes
- Swelling or the feeling of swelling (even if there isn't any)
- Rashes
- Dry eyes and/or mouth
- Dry skin
- Issues with coordination/balance
- Cramps in muscles
- Menstrual pain
- Pain or sensitivities with or after intercourse (muscular, higher sensitivities)

## <u>Diagnosis</u>

Fibromyalgia is one of those wonderful conditions that do not have a strong and definitive test. Usually with Fibro, the doctors have to rule out other possible conditions first. Once most other conditions (*Lupus, Lyme, CFS, MS*, etc.) are ruled out, then the doctor may do a "trigger point" test. This is when the doctor presses on 18 specific points on the human body to see the reaction. If a person responds strongly to 11 of the 18 trigger points, they are usually diagnosed as having Fibromyalgia.

Currently, though, researchers in Sweden and Australia are working on a blood test to be used to test for Fibro. This test finds a specific genetic marker that is similar to *Rheumatoid Arthritis* but slightly different. It is believed this marker may be the actual genetic tag for Fibromyalgia. If this is true, then future generations will have a much easier time being diagnosed without facing the ridicule and disbelief that many of us still have to deal with, as well as the constant tests and procedures used to rule out other possible culprits.

Fibromyalgia is considered a genetic disorder. The disorder affects more women than men at a ratio of about 7 women for every 1 man. The disorder also usually shows itself later on in life and is rarer to find in children. Doctors are still unsure of the exact cause of the issue or what sets it off. Currently, it is believe that traumatic physical or mental events, severe infections, and even slow build-up throughout one's life, lead to the activation of Fibromyalgia. I say "activation" because if you have Fibro, you were born with Fibro. It can lay dormant in a person until they die. Many more people possibly have Fibro but it has never fully manifested itself strong enough to become a problem.

Unfortunately, as the years have progressed, the prevalence of the disease is rising and the age at which it is active is dropping. More and more people at younger and younger ages are being diagnosed with Fibromyalgia. There is some concern that this has become a *SIDS*-like diagnosis. SIDS, or sudden infant death syndrome, was a term that referred to the unexplainable death of infants. The term is rarely used anymore because we now know that, most of the time, there is a reason for the death that is explainable. For a while, though, doctors used SIDS as a sort of "throw away" answer to cases of infant deaths that they could not figure out. Many people worry that this might be happening to Fibromyalgia. There is a possibility that with the use of the internet to research terms and symptoms and self-diagnosis, as well as the difficulty in proving the actual presence of Fibro, doctors use the diagnosis to either appease a patient that may be a hypochondriac or to try to put a name to a problem they can't figure out. This is unfortunate, as many of us still face the fact that other people think we are the *hypochondriacs* and that this is just "all in your head."

## Treatments

One of the harshest truths about Fibromyalgia is that there is no cure. There is also no one treatment that works for everyone, as well as no known treatment that completely helps with every symptom of the condition. There are prescription medications that help some people with some of the symptoms, lifestyle changes that can help with other symptoms, and over the counter medication that may help some people deal with the rougher days. All medications have side effects, many are very expensive and not covered by insurance, and there are always difficulties in changing your lifestyle to help cope with the condition. I will go further into the insurance issues and lifestyle changes later. Here I will cover a few of the more commonly used prescriptions, over the counter medications, and *homeopathic* remedies that some use to help them manage their Fibromyalgia.

### Prescriptions:

- <u>Lyrica</u> – (pregabalin) this drug is made to treat muscle convulsions/seizures and pain in people with shingles, epilepsy, diabetes, herpes, and Fibromyalgia. Side effects are swelling, weight gain, vision issues, and dizziness, drowsiness, and concentration troubles.

- <u>Cymbalta</u> – (duloxetine) the primary function of this drug is an antidepressant. It is also used for muscle and bone pain, but insurance usually considers it an antidepressant. The side effects are drowsiness and lightheadedness, sweating, swelling, weight gain, nausea, constipation, dry mouth and eyes, and loss of appetite.

- <u>Neurontin</u> – (gabapentin) this is considered a slow-release pain reliever used for muscles spasms and nerve pain. This medication can vary in doses from as low as 40mg up to 4800mg. The problem with the odd dosage is as it goes up, the amount of effectiveness can actually decrease. There have been studies showing that at a certain point, usually around 1800mg, the drug begins to lose some effectiveness. Side effects are vision issues, headaches, swelling, dry eyes and mouth, coordination issues, dizziness, drowsiness, constipation and/or diarrhea, weakness, and nausea.

- <u>Flexeril</u> – (cyclobenzaprine) A muscle relaxer used to treat pain, stiffness, and spasms in muscles. Should not be used if you are on *MAO inhibitors* or have any heart conditions or problems. Side effects include chest pain, elevated heart rate, headaches, drowsiness, numbness, weakness, nausea, and sensory issues. Can cause liver damage if you use it consistently over a long period of time.

- <u>Zoloft</u> – (sertraline) Medication used to treat OCD, anxiety, depressions, PTSD, and anxiety/panic attacks. Like most anxiety and depression issues, your doctor will usually start you on a low dose and work up, making sure to keep an eye on any adverse reactions, especially increases in anxiety or depression. It can cause dizziness, drowsiness, nausea, eye issues and headaches, and problems sleeping.

- <u>Effexor</u> – (venlafaxine) another anti-anxiety and depression medication. It also has been known to be used, on occasion, to lower pain issues as well. Side effects are drowsiness, stomach troubles, headaches, and dry eyes and mouth.

- <u>Prozac</u> – (fluoxetine) Anti-anxiety and depression, OCD, and bulimia medication. Side effects are drowsiness, difficulty sleeping, nausea and appetite issues, and possible sexual issues.

- Paxil – (paroxetine) An *SSRI* used to treat depression, anxiety, postpartum depression, OCD, PTSD, and panic/ anxiety attacks. Takes over a month to become completely effective. Side effects are drowsiness, vision changes, dry mouth and eyes, stomach problems, and sexual problems.

- Opioids – (Morphine, OxyContin, Tramadol, Methadone, Oxycodone/Percocet, Analgesics) Made from the Poppy plant, opioids are some of the strongest pain killers available. It takes a doctor prescription for each refill and is usually highly monitored. There are currently issues in the government and with the medical field in giving patients opioids as they are notorious for becoming highly addictive or for being abused by people who no longer or never did need them. Opioids cause drowsiness, confusion, blurry vision, stomach issues, constipation, dry mouth and eyes, itchy skin, sedation, growing tolerance, respiratory and heart rate issues, black outs, dependence, and even death if overdosed. Tolerance builds over time and causes the user to need more in order to get the same effect. An overdose can cause coma, heart failure, respiratory failure, vomiting, and death.

### Over the Counter/OTC

- Unisom PAIN – (contains acetaminophen) A sleep aid targeted at people with difficulties sleeping due to pain issues. One pill in a 24 hour period max. Causes drowsiness and sometimes headaches. I have a very high tolerance to medication and Tylenol, Motrin, etc. does nothing to help.

This can assist me if I am in moderate pain and really need to get a few hours of sleep, but that is my body and how it functions. We are all different.

- <u>Acetaminophen</u> – (Tylenol) Used to relieve pain. Overuse can result in liver damage and overdoses can lead to death.

- <u>Ibuprofen</u> – (Motrin) *NSAID* used to reduce fevers and swelling. Can cause stomach trouble, dizziness, and headaches.

- <u>Naproxen</u> – *NSAID* used to reduce pain, often not found very effective for people with higher tolerances to medication.

## <u>Homeopathic</u>

- <u>Melatonin</u> – Often used to help with insomnia. Causes drowsiness. WARNING: this should NOT be used on a regular basis if you have hormone issues, depression, anxiety, partial or full hysterectomies, or any other chemical imbalances. Melatonin is known to cause further issues with hormonal and chemical problems in the brain.

- <u>B12 Vitamins</u> – Vitamin often lacking in people without healthy diets and exercise. It is supposed to raise energy levels and help with memory and brain function.

- <u>Magnesium</u> – Used for energy, bone strength, and blood pressure regulation. Side effects can be stomach issues such as pain, gas, diarrhea, constipation, nausea, and vomiting if you consume too much or if you have issues with dehydration.

- <u>Vitamin C</u> – Used for energy and immune system health.

- <u>Omega 3 Vitamins</u> – Used for mood enhancement, arthritic pain, heart disease, and over all body health. Because it is often found in fish as well as plants, any signs of a allergic reaction need to be paid attention to. This includes difficulty breathing or swallowing, elevated heart rate, dizziness, coughing, swelling of face, and tightness in chest.

- <u>Vitamin D</u> – Used for the immune system, mood, and to strength musculoskeletal system.

**<u>Dietary Changes</u>** (Not for everyone, depends on other health conditions and ability to follow specific dietary changes. Talk to a healthcare professional before making drastic dietary changes. Also make sure to do your own research to see if a diet change is right for you.)

- <u>Gluten Free</u> – I have *Celiac Disease*. This means that I can't have gluten because my body has an autoimmune reaction that causes a lot of pain, distress, internal damage, mood changes, etc. I do know many people who have both Celiac and Fibro and haven't personally met someone with Celiac that doesn't have other issues like Fibro, CFS, or Lupus. This is probably because carbohydrates, in high and constant amounts, can cause problems in the body. So Celiac could be a part of a chronic pain condition. Health problems that cause nerve function issues that can affect organs would also be at risk for Celiac Disease (IBS, ICS, Fibro, MS, Lupus).That being said, I had a noticeable decrease in fog and flare days, headaches, rashes, and stomach issues when I did go to a gluten free diet. There is more about it in the section about my life story later in the book. This is a diet that cuts out anything made from wheat, barley, and rye. If you do not want to go completely gluten free, and I don't blame you for that, just cutting out excessive amounts of breads, cakes, cookies, crackers, breaded foods, pastas, and foods with artificial coloring and flavor (often made from gluten) can do wonders for your digestive system and health. Especially since these foods also have a high amount of sugar and saturated fat in them.

- <u>Sugar Free or Decreased Sugar</u> – This one isn't too hard to explain. Pure sugar is not good for your body. It tastes fantastic and I don't think I could go more than a few days without sweet tea, but it is really bad for you. If you look at many of the products you eat daily, you would be astounded at the amount of sugar in them. There are parasites in the stomach that live and thrive on sugar and has been noted to cause the "sugar addiction" that is known to plague Americans. You can research into this if you have a strong stomach and are not bothered by the little *candida* passengers we carry. Sugar also has no real nutritional value. Fruit alone provides more than enough for a person to consume on a daily basis. Many gluten free products make up for flavor by adding increased amounts of sugar and fake sugar is even more dangerous (especially with pain problems). A very popular hazelnut spread has a staggering amount in it! I was baffled when I read the label. The stuff is everywhere and leads to heart issues, diabetes, weight gain, vascular problems, and many other health issues. Reducing sugar is a great step for your health regardless of your medical problems.

- <u>Inflammatory Causing Foods</u> – There are many foods that have been shown to increase inflammation. The most common of these are what are referred to as "nightshade vegetables." The reason for this is the amount of pain and inflammation inducing chemical called solanine, an alkaloid that is related to arthritis pain. These vegetables are potatoes, tomatoes, eggplants, and many peppers (paprika, chili, bell, etc.).

- <u>Other changes to consider</u> – Depending on what issues you have specifically, will depend on what dietary changes can benefit you. Weight loss? Gluten free, sugar reduced diets, lower carbohydrates (starches like potatoes and pasta), and cutting out fried stuff can really help with preventing excess weight and giving your body better nutrients to raise energy levels, reduce pain, and get the proper nutrition you need. Stomach problems? It depends on the issues. If you have problems with constipation (opioids are a common reason for this), be careful with how much dairy, red meat, white rice, cheap junk food, and fibrous foods. With diarrhea related problems try to reduce the amounts of fruits, artificial sweeteners, fried foods, dairy, and gluten you consume. Gas and indigestion means less greens, beans, carbohydrates (potatoes and pasta), dairy, and fried foods. Another pain enhancing ingredient is aspartame, sugar substitute. This is found in "diet" drinks and sugar free foods and candies and is very bad for people with chronic pain. There are also some studies suggesting they may cause some forms of cancer.

- <u>DIETING</u>: If you are going to try any kind of diet, you need to make the changes small at first, and then slowly increase the changes. There are several reasons for this. First of all, slow and small changes can show you if what you are changing is helping or not as you remove or add a specific food. Second of all, sudden dietary changes can cause problems for the body if your body is used to eating a specific way. Drastic dietary changes could take you from having constipation issues to having diarrhea issues, or from gas to constipation. Sudden changes can shock the body and you need to be careful with this, especially if you start cutting out things your body actually needs. A good example is that fruit is a great source of many vitamins, but also may contain high amounts of sugar and acids. Fruits are great for most people but dangerous for diabetics or, if eaten in large amounts, people with digestive issues effected by acid (Chrohn's, ICS, IBS, etc.). Last of all, if you throw out everything you think is bad and tried to eat only the healthiest things you could, the cravings will get to you and you will binge and it will cause pain. Slow changes allow your body and your mind to adapt. Replace daily chip snacks with lightly salted caramel apple chips or lightly seasoned baked sweet potato chips. Instead of frying dinner, try baking it or cooking on the grill. You can get used to small and subtle changes, but big ones can cause you to revert back to old ways when everything is different and you are not used to the new tastes and textures. When I was first diagnosed with Celiac Disease, I had no choice but to make a major change to my diet. And once a month I would go and get a fast food cheese burger or a pastry and I would suffer for the next week or two. I missed those things and I didn't like the texture of gluten free bread and pastries. I hadn't gotten use to the changes so they were all new and not very pleasant. I wanted what I was used to, the flavors and textures I knew and liked, and I regretted it every time that want led to temptation. I haven't "cheated" by poisoning myself with gluten, on purpose at least, in almost a year and a half now. Though, often, it is very tempting.

## Therapies

- Hydrotherapy – This is the use of water to exercise or even just relax in. Because the water causes weightlessness, it helps take stress off of muscles, joints, and bones and can help people with pain conditions relax or even exercise without the painful impact that usually occurs.

- <u>Physical Therapy</u> – The use of forms of exercise and stretching to help strengthen muscles while being under the direct supervision of a physical therapist who knows your physical and medical limitations.

- <u>Meditation</u> – The use of mental relaxation to help ease stress, anxiety and depression, thus lowering pain intensity.

- <u>Massage Therapy</u> – Make sure you find someone that knows how to do massages on a person with Fibromyalgia or this can turn into a VERY painful experience for you. A proper Fibro trained masseuse can help relieve tense and knotted muscles and relax the body to ease the level of pain.

• • • •

## <u>Prognosis</u>

Fibromyalgia, itself, is not a fatal disease. It is, however, chronic. There is also a belief that, due to the issues that Fibromyalgia causes the nervous system and many other functions in the body such as sleep issues, temperature control issues, mobility problems, *and gastrointestinal* problems, people with the disorder have a tendency to end up with other health problems. There is also research in the growing connections between Fibromyalgia and other diseases such as Celiac Disease, Multiple Sclerosis, Lupus, heart disease and other neurological and autoimmune conditions. Many of the symptoms of Fibro are often related to, or can cause, other minor health issues that can escalate over time. A good example is the problems with IBS, nausea, and mobility can lead to issues with malnutrition, inability to absorb nutrients, issues with Type II Diabetes, and so on. Age can also play a factor. As you age, health issues can increase. Having a condition like Fibro already limiting your health and causing pain, the issue will only get worse as you age. It is inevitable and not a pleasant thing to look forward to.

This being said, one of the number one killers of patients with Fibromyalgia is suicide. It is a dark and sad truth, but one that has been recognized by several medical studies. There are several groups that help with depression and suicidal thoughts, including the National Fibromyalgia and Chronic Pain Association. As a person changes due to the limitations and the toll of pain and weakness to their body, it begins to show in relationships, jobs, hobbies, activities, and many other aspects of a person's life. Some people do not like even mentioning this and will probably complain about the fact that I did. Well, I warned you that I would be a bit more blunt about things than most people. This is not something that you can sugar coat. Being in several online social support groups, I have seen this come up in only the private ones where we are free to talk however we want. There are people and groups that require you to keep this "We can Make it!" or "Sunshine and Smiles, It could always be worse!" attitude. I get it, and yes, it most definitely could be worse. Honestly, though, I really get aggravated with the sunshine, bubbles, and puppies crap. I mean, good for you and all, but I am an "expect the worse so I am not disappointed and I get to be pleasantly surprised if it turns out even the slightest bit good" type of person. Pessimistic and negative, yeah, but I have been through a lot, and I am not going to get my hopes up or pretend to be that naïve.

We fake smiles all the time and pretend we don't hurt. You don't need to fake it with me. So, the truth sucks and hurts, but suicide is actually the #1 killer of Fibromyalgia patients. If you are considering suicide, if you even feel hopeless or depressed, reach out to someone, anyone. My information is at the end of this book. I have spent eight years of college focusing on psychology and I am a first-hand experienced person when it comes to black-out depressed and hopelessness. There are also lists of groups, websites, and other places you can check out. It sucks, it is not fair, it is not fun, and it can only get so much better, but there are others who have been through it. Read the section about me living with Fibro. Look at what I lost and the bottom I hit before I found my footing. "Big gentle hugs" is a common greeting and comfort phrase between people that suffer from chronic pain. I offer big gentle hugs, it isn't much but it is what I have to give other than this book.

## <u>Professionals and Fibro</u>

If you have been diagnosed with Fibromyalgia, then you have seen a doctor or three or ten. This can be one of the most stressful, aggravating, obnoxious parts about dealing with other people when you have Fibromyalgia. We are referred to as "professional patients." This is because Fibromyalgia is hard to diagnose. If we have reached the diagnosis, it has been through test after test, doctor after doctor, scare after scare, and more diagnoses than we can count. We have researched, studied, looked up, learned, and in my case I even took certification classes to know everything I could about our issues, inside and out. We have this crap down to a science, well, almost. But we need a doctor, and we need the help and the medications. So you go doctor hunting. Often medical professionals fall in one of several categories.

<u>Old school non-believers</u> – These are the professionals that got their degree back when Fibro was considered a mental issue. They haven't furthered their research or knowledge and will completely shut down as soon as Fibro is brought up. If anything, they know about Fibro but believe you have to be over 60, a woman, and crippled to have it. I have only known and met one person who started as an old school non-believer and changed her mind upon heavy research, arguments, testing, and persuasion. Thankfully, the numbers of these types of professionals is steadily dropping.

<u>Eastern medicine gurus</u> – These guys and gals are fun. They loathe Western medicine, believe everyone is a pill popper, and are pretty sure you just need diet, exercise, meditation, and sometimes even religion in your life to get better. They are usually a laughing stock and I have made a 180 and walked out of an office when a doctor immediately started spouting this rubbish. This is not saying that all "Easter medicine"

based medical professionals are this closed minded, but there is a very large group that is, so be warned.

Pill Pushers – These guys can seem like a blessing, they often don't ask questions if you tell them what you know works, and are pretty easy to deal with. The truth is, though, they are the reason we have so many problems trying to get opioid medication. I had one that seemed decent and respectable, though I thought it was odd that I could list OxyContin, Percocet, Clonopin, and Phenergan as my usual and "it actually works" medicines and he just wrote me a script with no questions. Unfortunately, on my disability case, I found out I could not use him for a reference because he was fired and arrested for giving lots of people whatever they told them, even though most didn't even have a doctor's order or a crate of medical files (like I carried around) proving need. They will give you whatever and then suddenly laws change, they get serious or close due to trouble, or they disappear and you are left without the meds you are used to and with a bad doctor on your record.

The hesitant-but-listening – These docs are the most common and can be difficult at first. You have to feel confident in what you are talking about, have your medical research and files in order, and believe in yourself. At first they may seem to not really trust your diagnosis, many even flat out tell you they do not believe you, but they take the file and say they will look it over or they will run a few tests to rule stuff out. It sucks, having the same tests done again and again, but it is worth it. Be confident and don't waiver. We call ourselves professional patients for a reason. We know what is up with our body and we went through the periods of confusion, tests, speculation, confirmation, denial, more confirmation, and then acceptance. We know what has happened and now they need to know. Stick with them, show them and teach them if they need it. In the long run, these have always been my best docs and PCMs. They realized I was correct and began to work with me in less than six months.

<u>The rare and elusive on-the-level</u> – This is a unicorn I have yet to see, but supposedly there exists these doctors that are up to date with the research and studies, that will read your file and believe that all your past docs and specialist are not liars, and they will immediately work with you. If you find one, put them in a golden cage and charge everybody to visit them during specially reserved viewing hours. And send me a free pass if you can.

## **<u>Docs who treat it</u>**

- <u>Rheumatologist</u> – A doctor who specializes in the musculoskeletal systems and autoimmune diseases. Often works with patients with arthritis, Fibromyalgia, Lupus, MS, and other conditions that need specific diagnostic criteria met in order to understand and treat their ailments. Usually considered the best doctor to go to for Fibromyalgia treatment.

- <u>Psychologist</u> – Doctors trained to work with a person's mental health. Usually helps through "talk therapy" in which you spend a specific amount of time at certain intervals with the doctor talking and focusing on issues that can be causing depression and/or anxiety as well as other mental issues.

- <u>Psychiatrist</u> – These are the same as psychologist with one difference, psychiatrist are doctors first and thus are allowed to prescribe medications, something a psychologist cannot do.

- <u>Physical Therapist</u> – A medical professional trained to help someone rehabilitate, regain muscle and body movement, and/or strengthen specific parts of the body in a regimen specified to the physical limitations and needs of the patient.

- <u>Pain Management Specialist</u> – A doctor who is allowed to prescribe patients with a multitude of medications, including opioids. Usually requires regular and sporadic urine testing and pill counts to insure the patient is not abusing any prescribed narcotics.

- <u>Neurologist</u> – A doctor who is trained and specializes on the nervous system and the nerves of the body.

## **Insurance and Disability**

I combined these two areas because they are very boring and dry, and the insurance is only going to be a small bit of information. Why? Well, insurance varies greatly depending on the type, the coverage, the specialist and doctors, and so on. So really I only have a few things I want to mention about that. Disability is not a big area as that too can have many variables, but there is some information I want to give you about trying to get disability. This information pertains to United States laws and may vary in other countries. I am unsure of procedures and policies in other countries. Any information is very welcome and could help me update future books on the subject.

<u>INSURANCE</u>

Getting insurance is difficult enough. With Fibromyalgia often being a "pre-existing condition," many insurance companies may make you wait from six months up to a year before treating the condition. Some private insurance companies are also known to deny patients with pre-existing conditions, so be aware of what the company you are trying to get allows. In the U.S., insurance has recently become a mandatory requirement. There is now a yearly fine if you have not had insurance for at least half a year and if you do not meet the low-income criteria. Many states do have programs that are provided for those who make under a certain amount a year. You can find out more about the programs through your county welfare, human resources, Department of Children and Families, or whatever it is called in your state.

Insurance will present two problems for you. The first will be trying to get a specialist and the second will be with prescriptions. Sometimes insurance may require you to get a referral, basically a permission slip, from your doctor to see a specialist. Other times they may allow you to pick a specialist in a specific area or off of a specific list. It is important to follow this protocol. If you need to see a specialist and your doctor, for some reason, is not giving you a referral, you can do one of two things. Either look for another doctor or contact your advocate in the insurance company. You need to have this on hand anyways. Almost every insurance company has an advocate or agent that works directly with you. This is someone or a specific number you can call about questions, any questions, when dealing with doctors, referrals, medications, etc. Call them and ask them what your options are. It is possible you may have to try to convince your doctor to write the referral or go through the hell of finding another primary doctor anyways. I suggest looking online and trying to find a site that lists Fibro friendly doctors. Ten years ago I would not have been able to find this information online, but with the difficulty of finding one, many people have banded together to make lists of doctors they know are Fibro friendly. Remember, you can give doctors interviews like you would if you were hiring an employee. A doctor is YOUR employee. You pay them, or you pay the insurance that pays them, or you paid the taxes that pay the insurance that pays them. Regardless, they work for you. You can make a list of doctors, call their offices, and say you would like to have a short appointment to meet and greet the doctor and see if they are right for you. You have the RIGHT to do this! Although many offices will still charge you a $20 or more fee to even see make an appointment.

The second issue is getting certain prescriptions. Some insurance companies do not cover prescriptions at all and you have to have a secondary company that does this. There are also options to get the reduced cost cards that allow reduced costs on some prescriptions but usually only the name brands and not generics. Another problem with prescriptions and insurance is how the insurance companies categorize some prescriptions. Cymbalta, for example, is often used for Fibromyalgia patients to help with several of the symptoms. Most insurance companies consider Cymbalta an anti-anxiety or antidepressant and may refuse coverage if they do not cover "mental medications." Always check with the insurance company. Sometimes insurance companies can allow you to use a medication for the "off label" uses. This means that if you are using Cymbalta to manage Fibromyalgia, even though it is considered an anti-depressant, the "off label" use for Fibromyalgia is something that can be covered as it is not the same condition with the same medical code. You may have to get a doctor's note explaining what "off label" condition the medication is being used for and then send that to your insurance company. Fun fact, Viagra is a male enhancement supplement to assist with erectile dysfunction even though the medication is actually a heart and blood pressure medication and erectile dysfunction is only an "off label" use of the little blue pill.

As for a pharmacy, make sure they accept your insurance, but know that you can shop around for a pharmacy too. Find one with the lowest price for the prescriptions you need. Walmart has a pretty low plan; the military pharmacies do as well. I am unsure if CVS or Walgreens has changed their plans, but they used to be quite competitive against the Walmart pharmacy. I also really liked how I could log onto the Walmart website, check available refills, order them to be ready for pick up or even to have them delivered, and you can even prepay a wallet to have prescriptions auto filled and prepared. Unfortunately, the small town pharmacies often do not have the $3 generic prices and may not have some of the more specialized medications. This may be different in your area. Again, shop around. Call them or visit or see if they have a website. A pharmacy is like a doctor, you are paying them in one form or another and so they are like an employee, interview and shop around. You do not have to settle for ridiculous prices or a place that never has your much needed meds in stock.

<u>DISABILITY</u>

This leaves us with disability. What a nasty dirty subject this is! First I want to mention handicapped placards. These are those blue signs you hang from your rear view mirror, or rear view mirror of the vehicle of someone who does drive you around, that say you are allowed to park closer instead of hiking a mile. This is actually received through your driver's license office. You get a form that your doctor fills out and you take that to the driver's license office and they issue the placard. I was stunned how easy this was to do! No disability babble required.

Now, onto the wonderful government fiasco that is disability. This is such a pain in the ass. It really is. I am actually on my ninth, 9$^{TH}$! attempt at getting disability. I have had three cases where I tried to hire lawyers but due to me not having a vehicle or going to their offices, they didn't participate and time ran out on me. Let me explain a few things about disability. There are TWO kinds of disability, SSI and SSDI. I am going to explain what each one is and who can apply for them.

<u>SSI</u>: Available to low-income people who have never worked or/and are considered low income. Usually people qualified for Medicaid and food stamps.

<u>SSDI</u>: Only available to people who have worked within the past five years and have worked enough to pay a specific amount of social security taxes to be able to draw from it. They go by a system calling this amount of time and money "work credits" and use an algorithm to see if you have acquired enough "work credits" to receive SSDI.

When you apply for disability, you will get sent more forms that need to be filled out and phone calls you will need to answer. If you do not have a current doctor and therapist and have not seen one in a while, they will be making an appointment for you to see a doctor and a therapist at a time and place they tell you. All papers they send you need to be filled out and sent back as soon as possible. If you cannot make an appointment, call and reschedule as soon as possible. Everything in disability is time sensitive. If you have not worked in the five years previously to having disability, your possible amount to receive is greatly diminished. Remember when you applied. Write it down, circle it on a calendar, do what you need to in order to remember. If you have to reapply, it must be after a certain amount of time from when you applied the last time. I believe it is currently at least six months that you must wait after your denial. You also must respond within 10 days to all calls and letters (this is the date the letter is dated, not when you get it). If you are denied, you have 30 days to appeal or go against their answer. When you appeal, you need to get a lawyer. The lawyer will help take it to court where they will present your case and the appeal and try to get the disability benefits. Most disability lawyers are pro bono; this means they do not get paid until you get paid.

Currently, as of 2016 in the United States of America, Fibromyalgia is not considered a "disabling" diagnosis. Spain has recently changed this, as have a few other countries. In the U.S. though, you have to prove disability based on other factors. I have yet to meet someone with Fibro that doesn't have a list of other conditions. You need to figure out what your most disabling condition actually is. They will not grant you disability if they believe you can sit at a desk or be a Walmart greeter. In order to be disabled you have to have conditions that make it to where you are unable to sit or stand for long periods of time, have difficulty using your hands and feet, have cognitive problems (concentration, memory issues, etc.), blindness, or a psychological condition. Any conditions you have that you are using for disability have to be something that will last at least six months or more. The Social Security guidelines say three months, but because of the time it takes to even get disability, I would suggest six months. If you broke your arm or leg, that is not enough to get disability.

Using a psychological issue can have some serious repercussions if you are not careful. Anyone with severe anxiety, depression, or other mental conditions can get disability if the condition makes it extremely difficult up to impossible for you to work outside of your home, around people, or in certain situations. If you have a condition that is this severe or worse, this also means you are accepting a certain level of incompetence. The downside of stating this to the government is that this can also make it clear that you are unable to take care of other people, including your children. If you are a single mom or one who spends most of their time alone with the children, this can cause issues with social services and can even result in the removal of your children from your home. In worst case scenarios, if your condition is considered to be something that can result in you neglecting, harming, or killing yourself, there is the possibility of being declared too unstable to remain in public. This could then lead to you being admitted to a psychiatric facility. I have not personally heard of this actually happening to someone, but it is something I was warned about when I was going through severe depression and anxiety and was home alone with my son a lot. Only now that his father has custody and I am admitting that I have a debilitating social anxiety issue, is my son safe because he is no longer in the home with me. I do not aim to scare anyone, but I do think you should be told of the possibilities of these situations. If you know you have a mental issue that can cause harm to your children and/or yourself, you should seek help. There are anonymous agencies, phone numbers, chat rooms, etc. that you can find that can help you, even if they are just a listening ear. Do not let your pride be your downfall.

There is a link to the Social Security Disability site under the support section of this book. Most questions can be answered by reviewing their site and checking through the help and FAQ sections.

You can also look to see the specific diagnosis they approve at https://www.ssa.gov/disability/professionals/bluebook/ listing-impairments.htm . It is also important to understand that on average, people applying for disability that do not have a fatal or completely obvious disabling condition are denied 2-5 times and are not granted disability until the case is appealed and taken to court by a disability lawyer. The process is daunting, exhausting, and upsetting. It can be very aggravating trying to prove to someone that you are unable to work. Especially when their initial approval or denial is based on a couple of questions, a few of your records, and the word of the random doctors they contact. If you end up having to see one of their appointed doctors and/or psychologists, it is even more infuriating. These people meet you for five minutes, ask seemingly random unrelated questions, do no testing, and then tell the government if they THINK you are disabled or not. I cannot count the headaches and cries I have had over dealing with this mess. I also can't put enough emphasis on how many times I wanted to just give up. You get tired, pissed, annoyed, and heartbroken and you just don't want to keep doing it to yourself. I have horrible memory problems now and they are surprised if I forget to call back or send a paper in? I have no vehicle and really can't drive much due to confusion, dizziness, and headaches I get when I drive, but they are surprised I can't make a random appointment they made for me with only a week notice of having made it? These are just more wonderful things about having Fibromyalgia, CFS, or any other "difficult to diagnose" and highly misunderstood condition.

Now that I have explained the basics and the medical information regarding Fibro, let me give you my experiences. I have had a whirlwind of a life, a roller coaster ride that would spin most people's heads. There have been ups and downs and flat plateaus of unchanging situations, but I always found my footing. I know that you may come from a wealthy or poor past, with better or worse current circumstances. You may have throngs of supporting people around you, or you may feel completely alone (even if you are not). I don't care where you came from or where you are going, I just want to show you that no matter what, you are not alone. Sometimes, that may seem like a lie, but believe me, there is always someone out there who has at least had a similar experience.

Remember, though, no one has experienced EXACTLY what you have. No one can definitively have had it better or worse because what is easy for one may be hard for another. We can't decide someone else's pain or depression is better or worse than our own. Yes, I am sure someone has had it worse than you, possibly. Yes, it is possible you had it way worse or better than me. This is my story, though, and it may be vastly different than yours or eerily similar. Regardless, I am going to open my world to you. I don't do this for pity, but to show you what I overcame to get where I am now. It is important to know that I ended up with many more health issues other than Fibromyalgia. Most people who have Fibro will often end up with other health problems. This is one of many reasons why the ability to live a full and happy life, or whatever you are able to do, will vary greatly between people.

## Life before Fibromyalgia

Whether we want to admit it or not, it is not uncommon to find yourself referring to two different versions of yourself. There is always the before and after. Often you will see memes or blurbs about not letting your disease define you. This is true, I am not Fibro and Fibro is not me. Regardless, there are two completely different people within me. So now I want to tell you about the girl that was, the one that existed before my limitations and procedures and massive change. To me, she died. I mourned her passing for a long time. It took a great deal for me to overcome my loss and embrace the birth of the new me, who I am now. Some people will be outraged at this and say that she didn't die, she just changed. That may be true, to an extent. My process, though, was to accept the death of the before and then grow into who I am now as a new person.

Physically, I was much stronger than I am now. Mentally, I was weaker because I had not been tested with some of life's harshest trials. I did have health issues as a child. I got infections easily, had insomnia and migraines, and (though I did not understand it at the time) I had anxiety issues stemming from overdoses of adrenaline pushing me into random fight or flight modes. Despite these issues, I was athletic, articulate, sharp minded and witted, and adventurous. I did cheerleading for the town while in elementary school. I was a Brownie in Girl Scouts, until I got kicked out for setting the troupe leader's daughter's hair on fire (I blame boredom at "camping" in their house, cooking s'mores over a gas burning stove, and the over use of hairspray on a mean girl's head meeting the concentrated beam of light filtered through a magnifying glass). My school grades were superb, I learned to read when I was four years old and was writing my first little poems and stories by second grade. I loved running in the woods, taking all day walks, climbing the Appalachian Mountains on family vacations, pretending I was a gymnast in the yard, and playing rough and violent forms of sports with my siblings.

In high school I joined the marching band and orchestra. I did volunteer work at the junior high and worked some summers at a nearby retirement community. I got to go to Hawaii with the marching band for a week. There was a several mile hike up an inactive volcano that I actually ran up and down and back up on! I had awesome grades in advanced classes, was pre-accepted to many colleges, and dreamed of getting into forensics with the Federal Bureau of Investigations ViCAP (Violent Criminal Apprehension Program) unit.

This is the basic run down. I grew up in a small town in Florida. My family was poor. Every sport or activity that my siblings or I got into was a huge effort of fundraising, family and friends helping out, or pure luck. My trip to Hawaii was due to me being able to make the initial nonrefundable $200 or so and someone else dropping out at the last minute. They couldn't be refunded, but I was chosen to go on their ticket. She may not ever read this, but I will forever be thankful to her and her family for that opportunity. Things got a little better later, when we were able to get a decent home and both parents were working. I moved out early due to family and personal issues, but continued high school and worked under the table to keep moving forward. I married young, worked full time, my spouse was in the military, and I was attending college in my spare time when I wasn't volunteering as a fire fighter at the local fire station.

Then I conceived my son. The pregnancy was difficult from the beginning. I was diagnosed with *De Quervain's tenosynovitis* in my hands, something similar to *Carpal Tunnel*, but runs primarily down the thumb into the tendons of the arm. I was *pre-eclampsic* with a resting blood pressure of 160/110, which is dangerously high. By my third trimester, I had difficulty standing for long periods without getting dizzy or blacking out. I was a borderline gestational diabetic. I stayed ill and was always extremely tired. I envied women that could do yoga or go jogging and walking while pregnant. My weight gain was ridiculous for my diet. I had weighed an average of 140 lbs. most of my life and was now tipping the scale at over 200. My spouse was deployed by my third trimester and I ended up having to temporarily move in with my grandparents a few hours away. With the military I saw a total of 13 different doctors throughout my pregnancy. This became a huge problem towards the end as only my primary care doctor could allow me to have a C-section and she was nowhere to be found when the time came.

My son was due in early January. In mid-December I began to have contractions. At the hospital, I was two centimeters dilated. They gave me pain medicine and medication to stop the contractions and sent me home to try to wait it out. I had an appointment on January 6th at the naval hospital. I knew I was not coming home without having my son. I was right. Unfortunately, I didn't realize what that meant for me and my child. My labor was over 29 hours in total. I was *strep B positive* (a bacteria found in many mothers that is only harmful to the baby) and needed antibiotics for a certain amount of time before I could give birth. *Penicillin*, unfortunately, was a big no-no for me. This meant they had to use several other lower level antibiotics to protect my son. I was also vomiting with nausea and having difficulty breathing. At one point, everyone had to leave the room and when they returned a while later, I was on oxygen. The mask dried out my nose and mouth painfully and I had to constantly remove it to vomit and dry heave. My son was stuck in the canal for a bit and the nurses didn't want me to push. I was stuck with an epidural several times, unsuccessfully, until they left the needle in at a random spot. This helped keep my right foot slightly numb for the remainder of the labor, but nothing else. I was physically torn open by the doctor and my son was ripped out by hand. This resulted in three large tears needing stitches for me (plus organ damage I would learn about later) and a *cerebral hematoma* (blood on the brain) and a broken clavicle (collar bone) for my son. He was rushed out in a plastic box and I was left, covered in my own mess, in the delivery room. I actually got up off the bed by myself and went into the bathroom to clean up. They even had food delivered to the room and my messy bed, but it took several hours before they finally moved me to my postnatal room. That is a much longer and crazier story for another day.

The next few months were hell. My spouse didn't come back from deployment until my son was nearly four months old. He missed the majority of the initial issues for the baby. Luckily, though, my little boy persevered. He did end up hospitalized at a prominent children's hospital in Jacksonville, Florida. He had initial problems with the cerebral hematoma, a blister on his penis from the umbilical cord clamp (they missed and caught his penis in it), and issues being able to digest breast milk and formula. As time went by, though, he recovered and got better and better. Unfortunately for me, my body would never be the same.

By the time I gave birth I weighed 245 pounds. This was on a diet of mostly gummy snacks, milk, water, and crackers. My appetite has always been atrocious, but the pregnancy took it to another level. I didn't spring back, in fact, I wasn't even healing properly. My stitches did not seem to want to heal, I was always in abdominal pain, and using the bathroom was becoming a nightmare. This is another super long story, but it would take a year of hell and many doctors and hospitals to get a grip on what was happening. I promise to give some of the fun stories in my bad and good doctor sections. Needless to say, I eventually discovered I had what was called full *pelvic prolapse*. The damage done during the late stages of my pregnancy and how my labor went (since the doctors outright refused to give me a C-section that probably would have slowed many of my health problems down and wouldn't have ripped my organs), was immense. Basically, my bladder, colon, vagina, and uterus had been ripped from where they were supposed to be and were now laying in the bottom of my pelvis fighting gravity. This led to some major surgery that resulted in my uterus and part of my intestines being removed. My bladder, vaginal cavity, and colon had to be rebuilt and stabilized with meat taken from my left leg. The surgery was a success, for the most part, and was done by an amazing team of doctors in Baltimore, Maryland (where we were stationed at the time). Thanks to the military hospital not giving me a C-section, I would never be able to have children again.

Then things got bad again. My back hurt a lot, and all the time. Eventually I started collapsing randomly and would be unable to sit up sometimes. This led to another batch of good and bad doctors, horrible hospitalizations, and terrifying insanity as I slowly went paralyzed from the waist down. A wonderful infectious disease specialist at one of the hospitals I was admitted too, saw my chart and read my case. As I was once again back home in pain, paralyzed, and with no answers, I got a phone call from her. She knew what was wrong and needed me to come in as soon as possible. Lots of crazy tests and procedures and she confirmed that I had *Osteomyelitis diskitis*, a rare bone infection in my spine. Apparently during the abdominal surgery, they had to stabilize my lower organs to my spine and the spine was nicked. This is not uncommon and was not the fault of the surgeons. That surgery was intense and had a lot of high risks. Blood loss and infection were known issues and I had both. I lost almost three pints of blood and had two put back in. This led to some other complications we will get to later, including anemia and iron deficiencies.

So now I had a diagnosis. I had a *PICC line* put in. This is like an IV that goes in the inside of your upper arm and the tube goes through your vein and all the way to your heart. Three times a day I had to flush the line and hook-up an IV drip (two in the mornings) of antibiotics for three months. This did not go flawlessly. At one point my home nurse forgot to put a type of valve on my line when she refreshed the set-up. Air ended up being sucked into my line and made their way to my heart giving me excruciating pain. I called an ambulance because there was a line going to my heart and my heart hurt and I was scared. They did a CT scan and found a massive air bubble in the right ventricle of my heart. The doctor told me, bluntly, that all he knew to do was have me lay on my left side and he would watch and wait. Normally, they would attempt CPR and pronounce me dead; due to hearts failing with that much air in them (ever watched "The Omen"?). So that was scary as hell. The term used was a right ventricular embolism. This resulted in a weakened state for my heart. In fact, because of both the blood transfusion and the heart issues, I can no longer give or receive blood without great possible danger to myself. I also ended up with a site infection on the PICC line. Eventually, though, the spinal infection was gone, but it did result in major damage in my lumbar region of my spine.

During all of this, I was having issues using the bathroom. Constipation was an issue, as was emptying my bladder. I spent a lot of time on liquid diets and having a *catheter*. I worked up to self-catheterizing, using a type I inserted when my bladder wouldn't empty. It did become easier to go, but if I held it too long or if my back was hurting, I had to self-cath. This led to another wonderful hospitalization as I began to descend into kidney failure from an infection stemming from catheter use. I also got another PICC line then. Needless to say, I saw lots of doctors and hospitals and medications and my problems seemed endless.

While I was fighting for my health and even my life at times, one of my primary doctors was curious at my inability to heal enough for the pain to recede. I also began getting other weird symptoms. Many were initially believed to be related to medication, being a new mom, my other health issues, and (as one crappy doctor said) my ability to "imagine" pain in my belly "blossoming" to my body. There were some problems that didn't fit, though. Some being the feeling of spider webs on my skin or feeling like I had sunburn and that I was covered in sand. My brain was dulling. I couldn't think sometimes or form the words I was trying to think about. My memory tanked, I mean, it went bad! I couldn't remember what I was doing, where I was going, what I was supposed to be writing in college. Yes, I was still trudging through college via the internet and a lot of medical leave breaks. Sometimes I would feel random burning sensations, sometimes my joints would be excruciating, and my insomnia was worse, as was my migraines. I just felt awful, all the time. My primary doctor did a ton of x-rays, scans, blood work, and other procedures and tests. Then one day she asked me to lay on my stomach on the table, knowing it was not a comfortable position for me. She asked me to respond to her touches. Then she started poking me and I must have looked like a jumping bean. I jerked and gasp at every poke. She told me that she was pretty sure, in ruling everything else out, that I had Fibromyalgia.

The next few years were healing from one thing and dealing with ten other issues. I kept pushing. I went through depression, I wanted to give up. I would get renewed strength and push again. As I have mentioned before, Fibromyalgia is believed to be genetic. It is also believed you are born with it but often it takes a traumatic or severe illness or situation for those crossed wires to make their first spark. My rough pregnancy and difficult labor, coupled with the damage and surgeries afterwards, was very traumatic to my body. My doctor said it was more than enough to trigger the dormant disease. Through medical evaluations and family history, it is believed I inherited it from my mother, who inherited it from her mother. This can happen to men, and can be passed through men. For some, reason, though, it is mostly a female oriented disease. I have since been re-diagnosed two more times by skeptical doctors as having fibromyalgia. There is belief it may be something more severe, such as *Lupus* or *Multiple Sclerosis*, but those tests have always been inconclusive.

Despite the diagnosis, it was somewhat of a relief to find out I had a connecting issue that answered many questions and proved the pain and problems were not in my head. Something that made all the filler problems, in between my other health issues, makes sense. I would learn about *flares* and *fogs* and the changes that would occur living a life with Fibromyalgia. And so I did, and I studied and learned (both by studying and through harder routes of experiencing). I had to make adjustments, and then I had to make more adjustments. I wouldn't be putting out fires or climbing volcanoes. The biggest hit, the hardest hit, was the decline in my schooling and the changes my "dream job" underwent. I sacrificed and then I lowered my standards and then I lowered them even more and sacrificed even more. I reached some of my lowest lows and some of my bounces back up were not very significant. It took time, pain, understanding, acceptance, heartache, and a lot of changes to get to where I am now.

## Life with Fibromyalgia

For a recap, I had been diagnosed with De Quervain's, Fibromyalgia, insomnia, migraines, anxiety, and depression, damage to my spine from the infection, ICS, and IBS. I was also diagnosed with *degenerative disc disease, anemia,* iron deficiency (but I was also intolerant of iron supplements), *peripheral neuropathy, plantar fasciitis, vertigo,* ovarian cysts and so many other issues. So I was a mess. My spouse at the time was in the military still when I was diagnosed with Fibromyalgia and throughout all the other diagnosis and surgeries. He then became a truck driver. During those years, I actually didn't see him very often. For the most part, it was just me and my son unless I was having surgery, then a relative would visit to help out.

Things went bad, eventually, really bad. I was in the hospital with the kidney failure when one of our two vehicles was towed and we got a notice that we were losing the house. We packed up and moved to the foothills of the Smoky Mountain in Northern Georgia where a friend had a place we could stay. Things continued to fall apart. We moved into a shack on the mountain for a while. It was hard. In the winter it got cold. One year it was in the negatives. The pipes would freeze and I would have to travel to a nearby stream to get water and climb under the house to try to fix what I could. My spouse would be home about a weekend a month. I plan to write another book going more into the nitty-gritty parts of my life. So I am going to skim over most of that. I did, however, begin to have another issue. I coughed and vomited A LOT. I mean a gulp of water and I was coughing until

I vomited. I began getting bad chest pain, sharp pains. The emergency room was no help. Eventually they diagnosed me with *Costochondritis*, basically arthritis of the chest cavity. The pain continued, the vomiting continued, and so I started to eat less and less. I have to mention that at this point I had food stamps until my spouse began to get decent work as an over-the-road truck driver. So groceries weren't too big of a deal. I also, though, never really had a good appetite and nausea had always been a problem for me. The vomiting was starting to get out of hand. I was also still weighing in at 230-250 pounds, fluctuating by ten pounds every week. I wasn't eating much, and I was throwing up a lot, so why wasn't my weight dropping? I ate Tums and other antacids constantly. I was usually afraid to eat too much of anything.

I finally got an awesome doctor; well technically she was a nurse practitioner. I will write a bit more about her in my "Good Doctor Stories." She referred me to a specialist in *gastroenterology*. Then it was more tests. At this point, I had undergone so many procedures, nothing was really new. Previously I had surgery on my right hand for the De Quervain's, a test that checked my bladder and urethra by filling me with water while I sat in a toilet seat thingy above the doctor's and had my lady parts shocked until I peed myself, air sprayed into my bladder and biopsy's taken out, colonoscopies (tubes and cameras up my bum while I was unconscious), defecating proctogram (you get filled by a caulk gun looking thing with a paste up your bum that you then defecate out into a bucket in front of an x-ray machine), x-rays, CT scans, bone scans (injected with radiated stuff and scanned while you lay on a metal table and your bones glow green on the screen where breaks and infections are), MRIs, urine tests, blood tests, and so on. So more tests did not surprise me, but it was the first time I would have tubes and cameras down my throat (while unconscious, thankfully). They discovered my stomach was up in my esophagus because the esophageal colon, or little muscular door, between my esophagus and stomach had stopped working. If I bent over, my stomach and the contents would flow out. It was a hiatal hernia. The answer? They had to go in and pull my stomach down to where it should be and wrap over half of it around the base of my esophagus so that when my stomach contracted, it closed off the esophagus. Good news was no more vomiting and stuff coming out and less chest pain. Bad news was I could no longer vomit or burp and my stomach could now only contain 1/3 of what it could before. This worked for a bit, but I still was having problems eating.

I was eventually sent to a surgeon who discovered my gallbladder had become completely diseased in the matter of a year. On top of this, I had crazy sores all over my legs, back, butt, stomach, face, neck, etc. I was still swollen and not losing weight. The gallbladder was removed. My primary doctor then decided that the damage to my intestines pointed to a very logical possible problem. I had *Celiac Disease*. She told me to cut out all gluten from my diet. Gluten is an elastic molecule found in wheat, barley, and rye. Unfortunately, this little molecule in used in EVERYTHING. Anything artificially flavored or colored usually contains gluten: caramel color or flavor, most breads, crackers, cookies, noodles, canned goods, boxed goods, pre-seasoned stuff, etc. It is in so much stuff! I went a week without it. This was crazy for me. I didn't eat much, but when I did eat it was toast or some crackers. Now I couldn't have that. Even spaghetti sauce often has it in there, as gluten is often used as a thickener for seasonings and sauces. So fruits, vegetables, meats I seasoned with spices and such that was not premixed (season salt has gluten in it), and dairy products that were actually dairy and not "products" (cheese "products" like sliced cheese has gluten in it). The sores started to disappear, the nausea lessened, the constipation and diarrhea back and forth got less and less. I am a hard head. I said "bullshit" and ate a few cheese crackers and a short bit later I had a headache, my stomach hurt, and several other issues started acting up. So I stopped again. After a month and more testing, it was confirmed. I had Celiac Disease.

After that diagnosis, things sort of evened out, at least on the surface. The truth was that I spent most of my time lying on the couch. The medications made me lethargic, nauseous, and out of it. My mentality was a mess. My spouse and I argued often. When he was home, he would find reasons to be gone the whole two days he had off. I had given up so much. It killed me to watch my little boy play and I was too tired and in too much pain to play with him. College suffered. I went from straight A's to C and D's. I had taken off so much time for medical leave and they knew of my diagnoses. I had gotten my A.S. in Criminal Investigations and had been working on an excelled program to get my Master's in Neurological Psychology and Forensic Psychology. The harsh truth was I would never be a detective, never an FBI agent; I couldn't even work in behavioral sciences with the FBI. I probably couldn't even be a psychologist at this point. The government believed this too and offered to pay off my student loans if I agreed to no longer continue my course of studies and agree I was medically unable to get a job in the fields I was studying in.

Somedays I could function to a point. Those days I would sit outside and watch my son play, I would play my violin or cello or clarinet, I would watch a movie or read a book or play a video game. I would sometimes craft soaps and lotions or design and sew clothing. Other days I could barely think. I couldn't focus on the television or on a book. I could barely sit up. I wanted to die. I wanted to send my son to my family in Florida and die. It did not help that my spouse began joking about replacing me, about me training a replacement wife for when I did die. I was at a high risk of colon cancer because of the damage to my gastrointestinal systems, ovarian cancer because of my ovarian cysts, leukemia and blood cancers due to my issues with that, infections because of my terrible immune system and the problems I had with my kidneys and liver. I felt like I was dying, I wanted to die. My son was the only thing that kept me from killing myself. I thought about it when I took my medication (always taking less than prescribed due to having people in my family having drug abuse issues). I thought about it when I saw my gun. I thought about it too much. My support was absent. My spouse and I were two different creatures by then. I wasn't the girl he fell in love with and he was always gone. He never fully doubted me, but he had done a lot of awful things showing his lack of interest or care. That is more dark stuff for my personal story but that is a different book.

So lots of personal stuff happened that led to me and spouse separating. I met an awesome guy in the one way I refused to ever meet anyone, online. He talked to me for hours and hours. He didn't care about my health issues and was perfectly fine with me having a child. In fact, when I told him that my son was a large portion of my life, he admired my dedication and told me he wouldn't expect less. He didn't care that I was overweight and scarred all to hell and back. He thought I was intelligent and strong. We connected on more levels that I could imagine, though neither one of us was actually looking for a relationship at the time. I also made another radical, and very dangerous, change. Let me warn you, never EVER stop your medications cold turkey. You need to wean off of them, and even then you should have a doctor working with you on that. I lost my insurance and my doctors and my prescriptions with the separation. In fact, I would have been homeless if not for the man that would be my future partner. He took in me and my son (though my son spent a lot of this transitional time with my brother a few hours away and my mom in Florida). I stopped everything. All my medications got flushed. I started smoking marijuana on a regular basis. This is not for everyone, I know. Everybody has their stand and their reasoning, I do not judge. For me, it worked. When I had marijuana I could sleep, eat, and was more relaxed. Without it I stayed awake up to four days at a time, went days without eating, was always nauseous and had headaches, and the pain was worse because I was stressed.

The problem was, no matter what, I still had bad days. I still could not function. I also lost the vehicle I had at the time with the separation. I had no way to work and if I did, no one would hire me. The jobs I tried didn't like my weight lifting restrictions and inability to be able to always come in. I had dietary restrictions, I was unable to be around certain products (food isn't the only thing with gluten in it), I couldn't stand or even sit in the same position for long periods of time, and I got headaches and dizzy spells a lot. I could barely afford to feed me, much less my son. More personal drama and a lot of bullshit, but my ex was moving back to Florida with to my family. We decided, along with my son, that my son should go with him. They were going to provide food, shelter, and help my ex get back on his feet. It was messed up and really crazy, but if they were going to take in my ex then they could help him take care of my son, even if they refused to help me.

And so I said bye to my baby not knowing when I would see him again. It crushed me. I stayed dark and locked in myself. I cried until I was dehydrated and my face was swollen and raw. I hated my family, my ex, and myself. There was a lot of misunderstanding. I was the type of person that kept personal problems personal. My family never knew of the things my ex did, they never knew of how he acted, the things he said, and so on. He got to my family before me and spun a beautiful story of me doing drugs, living in a whore house, and all sorts of insanity. I was almost impressed, since I spent my time at my partner's dad's house, usually watching movies or reading, maybe playing games or sewing. I smoked weed, cigarettes, and drank sweet tea....oh the horrors of my ways! I was so disgusted, so angry, so hurt, I didn't care. As long as my son was safe, happy, and healthy, I didn't care what they said about me. My son is brilliant. He is nine now and so very intelligent. This was a little boy who explained the molecular structure of fire to my brother when he was five. I told him to always be himself and not what others wanted him to be, to always think his own thoughts and to tell people to "shut up" if they said things he didn't like hearing. I told him to call my partner's phone whenever he wanted to talk to me. I gave him phone numbers, email addresses, even made a skype account, everything that he could carry around to contact me if he needed too. I talk to him every week, though there has been a week or two where I am unable to. I only get to talk to him when he is visiting my mother, whom I have rebuilt trust with and worked through a good bit of the drama. I am extremely happy that she and I were able to regain the bond we had before. My son lives with his father and his father's girlfriend a bit south of my mom. Luckily, though, my son is with my mom at least once a week or more, so we can talk.

Needless to say, I hit a bottom I had never hit before. I really wanted to die then. Why not? My son was safe, I had no home or job or anything, and my partner and I weren't official yet (we were kind of friend's with benefits). Things began to change though. I was in support groups and one of them was a private group of 29 women. After a few months we were 27. Two of the women committed suicide. Both had never shown signs or were outwardly depressed. Like me, they were holding it in, sitting in the dark somewhere, occasionally making a quip or two online and secretly dying in their own minds. On top of that, my partner and I were becoming serious. He had already changed his life plans a month after meeting me when he moved away like he planned and I stayed in his old room and helped his dad out like I planned, but then I missed him and he missed me and things weren't working out and so he came back. He was there while I came off all my meds, he was there while my ex created madness and heartache with my family, and he was there holding me when I cried for a week or more straight at the absence of my son. Some people ask why he didn't get a better job and help us or do more. That pisses me off. We weren't sure what would happen between us. I could have picked up and went to Florida to try to work things out. I could have died or killed myself doing something stupid. My son was not his child to take care of. It wasn't his place or responsibility to drop everything and try to get a better job and life for a disabled woman and her child that he had only known for a few months. He beats himself up over it anyways, but it wasn't his responsibility. So screw those who felt the need to judge someone that had shown me and my son more care, concern, and help than anyone else had.

My partner was supportive, understanding, and helped me realign myself to what I needed to be to move forward in life and not end it in some dramatic overthought style. It is amazing the difference one person in your life can cause. Yes, I still hurt and my body was always being a pain in the ass, but I had reasons to push through. I had someone who loved my cooking but didn't complain when I didn't feel well enough to cook. He admired my clothing I made, the ceramics I painted, the lotions and soaps I would make, but he never complained about the space my materials took or how much time lagged between projects or that I didn't make a whole lot of money doing them. He supported my writing and was appreciative of what I could do. He supports me staying in contact with my son and hopes to help me get in a situation where, if my son wants, he could move back with me. I had never had anyone give me that much without me giving my all. Yes, he has his faults and can be a major pain in the ass. Sometimes, he even says the wrong things to deal with my anxiety attacks or fears about my health, but nothing like I hadn't gotten from people who supposedly cared much more for me. But for the first time ever, I had someone come into a dark room where I was crying and hating the world and myself and he would just sit by the wall, waiting until I was ready for comfort. When I would finally calm down he would hold me and comfort me. He isn't perfect, but I honestly believe he saved my life and with two years under our belt, he is pretty damn perfect for me.

My ex has refused to sign divorce papers on many occasions for miscellaneous reasons. I hear he is expecting a child soon, so maybe I will finally get that divorce. I talk to my son often and he is supposed to be coming to spend the summer with us. My biggest change is what you are reading right now. I have wanted to write a book since shortly after I began reading. I have started so many books. Most are fantasy or horror fiction that I get ¾ of the way through and then lose interest or read something similar and I give up. I have written poems that have been published. I have ghostwritten books that other people have been published under their name. Granted most of those are cheesy romance or smut books I wrote because I needed the money. This is my first book though; my first "breaking into print." I have given so much advice to other people and explained so much to people that I decided to write about it. I am also currently writing a book that is a collection of short eerie and psychological thriller type stories. I do plan on continuing this line of writing as well, though. I plan to write a book about Celiac Disease and possibly some on depression, anxiety, insomnia, etc. I want to give people a casual and blunt dose of information. I like helping people and I am hoping this book does actually help a lot someone. If I do well enough, I can probably stop writing the crappy books under other peoples' names and get my own name out there. I want to beat the odds. It has been a hard and difficult journey. I have actually, seriously, nearly died on several occasions; kidney failures and breathing failures and suicide attempts when I was a teen (not including thoughts of suicide as an adult).

I am here now, though, and I want to be here for you. I promise, someone, somewhere, will listen to your story. Someone will be your shoulder. And if you don't want anyone or any shoulders, that is fine too. Fibromyalgia sucks and it is the crux of most of my problems, but it is not me. It is merely a reason why I may not write any tomorrow or why I am writing this in the first place. As terrible and frustrating and scary and alone and tired and achy this disorder makes me, it has allowed me to write this for you and others like you. I have found some small modicum of peace. And that, my friends, is the short version of my story.

## Good Doc Stories

*A tale of two hospitals part A:* This is in two sections because I was taken to the county hospital first and after four or five days, transferred to the big medical center for a week. The county hospital was amazing, the medical center was not. I had to call the ambulance because I had fallen, due to inability to use anything below my mid back, twice the night before and then down the stairs in the house the next day. My spouse did not seem too concerned so I called an ambulance to come get me. This was in Maryland, and they took me to a small county emergency room nearby. That trip sucked. Every bump in the ambulance was torture. They got me there and everything was blurry for the next few days. The pain and back spasms were excruciating. They had to catheterize me and hooked me up to IVs. I was given morphine and two hours later diluadid and two hours later morphine and back and forth to try to keep me from causing more damage when I had a spasm. Every time one of those painful spasms would hit, though, my body would arch up in the middle of my back causing more pain.

I had at least two nurses checking on me. Once a day I was given a sponge bath in the bed. The doctors were scrambling trying to find out what was wrong. This was the hospital where that amazing infectious disease specialist saw my file and called me later believing she knew what I had, and she was right. She had been there, coincidently, because another one of her patients was in the ER. They did all they could, but they did not have the equipment and specialist to find out what was going on with me. Since I had my recent major surgery in Baltimore, they wanted to send me back to that hospital so my surgeons would be available to get on the case and find out what happened or went wrong. Their intentions were pure, they took great care of me, the staff was so sweet, and I really wish I could have stayed there. Once the next ambulance took me to Baltimore, everything went downhill fast. The other half of this story continues in the "Bad Doctors" section.

*A special kind of specialist*: This one is kind of short because I have mentioned her a few times already. This infectious disease specialist happened to be at the right hospital and at the right time for me. She was at the ER checking up on another patient when she overheard staff discussing my case and trying to figure out what to do. She got enough information to get the basic idea of why I was there, but not much more. That hospital did run some x-rays, but nothing substantial had shown up. I am unsure if she asked for more information there or just followed my case, but after the hell I endured at the next hospital, I left in a hurry against doctor's orders via a wheelchair. When I checked my messages, I had received a phone call from this doctor. She apologized for knowing about my case and not being my doctor, but she said she had a pretty good idea what was wrong and I needed to come see her immediately.

I went to her office, hours were almost over, but she was in no rush. She had gotten my permission to get the x-rays and had them. She ran a blood test and scheduled a bone scan the next day when she knew she would have my results. I came in for the bone scan, and that was crazy. You get in a gown, lay on a metal table, they bring out a weird injection needle in a metal syringe that is still steaming from the cold thingy they pulled it out of. It was put in my IV and the bone scan began its work. It was kind of neat. I was able to watch the screens as it scanned me. She freaked out on my left foot, which I had forgotten I had broken before my major surgery and did not fully heal by the time they had to remove the cast for the actual surgery. So my left foot began glowing bright green on the screen. My lower spine was also glowing, and not in a neat "spine shape." She then took me to her office and explained what had happened. She said my spine had been nicked by a scalpel or needle during surgery and it had gotten an infection in the bone. This was causing swelling, degradation to the bone and discs, and nerve damage. She put me on the intravenous antibiotics and placed a PICC line in my arm. That was another crazy experience. You lay on a table under a live x-ray and watch the screen as they push the tube in your arm and you feel a cold sensation moving along with the path of the tube on the screen, until it is in your heart. It was crazy to watch that.

She saved the day again, later, when a nurse tried to give me the wrong antibiotics, something that would probably kill me if it went into my heart, as it was a form of Penicillin. They had the bag hanging next to me, went to go get something before hooking me up and she came by, checked the bag and panicked! That nurse got her ass chewed out for not cross checking files and labels. Although, she was trying to reduce my IV bags to two a day instead of 4-5, but she did not check my chart to see why I had to get a different medicine. The doctor kept checking my IV over the next few months and was the one to notice the slight discoloration and had an immediate blood test done when she suspected the site was infected. She was prompt, intelligent, nice, and really good at her job, this short, young doctor from India, the woman who saved me from permanent paralysis and death (once the infection travelled up my spine and into my heart). She was really amazing.

*Two of a kind; sincere surgeons*: When I discovered, after some intense internet searching, that the weird issues I was having when I went to the bathroom was actually my organs trying to escape my body, I was terrified. I eventually did further research and found a doctor in Baltimore who was rated one of the top prolapse surgeons in the United States. I made an appointment with her and took the journey to see her. The procedures and tests she put me through were not fun at all, many were humiliating. In fact, this was where I first had the test where they inject water into your bladder, sit you on a toilet seat shaped thingy, raise you to about head level for them, hook up some electrodes to your girl parts, and then send random electrical waves (that you can't really feel) to see when your bladder gives out. Once she did her initial tests, she was baffled. She told me that before me, the worst case she had seen was a 27 year old (I was 22 at the time) who had pushed a pickup truck about twenty feet and caused the muscles to tear inside giving her bladder and colon prolapse. I was much, much worse. She had to call in another surgeon because she was only an uro-gynecologist and worked only with the female reproductive system and bladder. In comes my gastroenterologist surgeon.

Together, they started making the plan on how to help me. The GI surgeon is the one that initialized the defecating proctogram, the caulk gun up the bum and then poop in front of an x-ray. They discussed options with me. The first was whether I wanted another child or not. If I did, I need to try to conceive immediately, I would probably have to be hospitalized, the baby would have a 30% survival rate and I would have a 60-70% survival rate. I already had my son who was just over a year old. I could not risk him losing his mom or nearly dying to have a baby that would not make it and cause me more heartache. On top of that, my spouse was not happy about us getting pregnant the first time and had no interest in having another child. So it was decided, my uterus would be removed. Due to the extent of prolapse in my colon, part of my intestines would also have to be removed. They would then have to suture and reconstruct my colon, bladder, and vaginal cavity and then use a sling to hold them in the right place. The sling would be attached to my spine. They wanted to know if I wanted a synthetic sling or one made from my own muscle tissue. The synthetic sling was still new and had some dangers attached to it. The body could reject it, the possibility for infection was higher, and it could degrade over time. I decided to go with the sling made from my muscle. Good thing I did, less than three years later those synthetic slings were recalled due to infections and rejection issues.

The meat had to come from my leg, we decided the left leg. They had to open me up through a slit on the side of my leg a few inches above the knee and it would be about six inches long. The meat was about 6x18 in size and would be taken from my whole thigh. They also had me come back twice to donate blood for myself as bleeding was a major risk in the surgery. I had stitches from the back to the front, inside my vaginal cavity, and up my thigh and staples from hip to hip.

It was a lot of work. These ladies were always good natured, welcoming, asking about my son and how I was doing, always remembered me and my son's name, and all around really great bed side manner. They had a lot of work and did a great job. There was a lot that could have gone wrong. Some women are unable to have sex due to pain after this procedure. Sometimes the stitching is too tight and the vaginal opening could be too small for sex or the stitched area inside could have nerve damage and you are either unable to feel at all or it hurts. There are also bowel issues that can come from it. Sometimes the colon is not done properly and the rectum will not open right for a bowel movement or you could have anal leakage from it not closing all the way. Muscle and never damage could make you unable to properly have a bowel movement and could lead to the need of a colostomy bag, a bag that has a tube that goes into your stomach for your body to send waste too instead of having a bowel movement. I do have difficulty with using the restroom, but it is not nearly as bad as it could have been. They did a wonderful job and constantly called to check on me. They took every concern seriously and were very thorough. I was really happy that I found them to do such a delicate and dangerous procedure.

_Elder professionals can learn new tricks_: A former primary care manager of mine was a nurse practitioner. She worked for the doctor who was technically my doctor, but whom I have never met. Overflow patients see the nurse practitioner instead of the primary doctor at this particular clinic. This concerned me a bit from the beginning. I was supposed to see this doctor, not the nurse that helped her around the office. Well, I quickly realized that wasn't exactly what was going on. The nurse practitioner was my doctor, she worked just as well as someone who had that title, and there was little to nothing that she couldn't do as my primary care physician that a doctor could do. Apparently this is common practice in many decent doctors' offices, so that the doctor is running the office and can have more patients then they normally could see, but each patient would still get good individual care. And I did eventually talk to the doctor on a few occasions if anything came up, as she would contact me directly and work out what the nurse practitioner would need to do next.

Anyways, so my first appointment with my nurse practitioner was not wonderful. The woman was in her late forties to mid-fifties range, had been a practicing nurse for over twenty years, and walked in with a stern and skeptical expression on her face. I was in my mid-twenties, weighed about 245 pounds, wore frumpy clothing, and had a box of files with me. The first thing she said, after introducing herself, was "You're too young to have Fibromyalgia. Women with Fibromyalgia are at least fifty years old." I didn't say anything, I waited for her to scan down my paperwork some more. She saw my list of surgeries and asked for more details about the procedures and what happened afterwards. I filled her in the best I could, using my handy notebook (where I had been keeping a timeline from my pregnancy on of every ER visit, hospitalization, doctor appointments, illnesses, surgeries, and anything else I could remember or find and write down and once you start filing for disability, having a timeline with all this information written down will save your brain and a lot of aggravation).

She was concerned about my weight, but also concerned about my pain issues and nausea. This was before I was diagnosed with Celiac Disease (which ended up being her who discovered that one) and my gallbladder was still in. I hadn't found out about my stomach being in my esophagus or any of that. She ordered blood work, a urine test, and an x-ray. We set up another appointment for a week out. I came back and she was a bit warmer and polite, not as cold or stern. She said my blood results showed inconclusive for Lupus and rheumatoid arthritis. My blood results also showed I had no bad cholesterol, but I also had no good cholesterol. This was the first proof that there was something going on other than me sitting around, being lazy, and pigging out on junk food. My white blood cell count was high, my sugar levels were normal, and my blood pressure was normal. In the first two months, she ended up prescribing me Zoloft for my anxiety and she refilled my Phenergan for nausea. She also started me on Clonopin again to help me sleep and deal with my anxiety attacks, which I had been unable to get for a few months while in between doctors. She still wasn't 100% certain about the Fibromyalgia diagnosis, even though I had been diagnosed by two different doctors at two different points in the last five years.

Reluctantly, I printed out a bunch of information about Fibromyalgia as well as my charts from Patients-Like-Me (a great place to keep track of your medications, medical history, treatments, conditions, daily symptom logs, moods etc.). I brought them to her and apologized for being forward or assuming she did not know any of this, and I gave them over. The next appointment, she did the tender spot test and she nodded, apologized for her initial reactions, and concluded I did in fact have Fibromyalgia. Over the next few months, she began to really open up. She helped me find good doctors and get procedures down to deal with my stomach, esophagus, and gallbladder problems. She figured out the Celiac Disease, I hadn't even known what that was. Within less of a year of meeting her, she was asking my permission to have students sit in on our appointments. The first time she did this she told the student "Now, with this one, throw your book out the window. Her issues, past, and symptoms are kind of crazy, but this girl knows what she is talking about, so listen to her."

It broke my heart when I moved and she was no longer my primary care doctor. I really loved how well we worked together the last year I was with her. She tried physical therapy but halted it when my spine was in danger. She refused to put me on sleep medication because she took the side effects of black outs and sleep walking seriously. She helped me get decent pain management services and helped me work through other medical issues. I stuck with her, even though our initial appointment seemed like a bad omen. I am glad I did and I hope to find another doctor like her one day.

## **Bad Doc Stories**

*A tale of two hospitals part B*: So, in the previous section, part A of this, I told you about the amazing quality of care at the county hospital. This is what happened when the ambulance I left in, reached the main surgery center in Baltimore. I was taken to the ER, or so I was told. I was mostly out of it due to the pain medicine and sedatives they had given me in order to make a two hour ride with my back spasming, buckling, and hurting. Apparently, for some reason, from the ER I was taken to one of the other four towers of the facility that kept the Emergency Room inpatients instead of the tower where my surgeons had their inpatient rooms. This meant, my surgeons and doctors, were not informed of where I was. I would find this out much later. The rooms were pea green, two beds, two televisions, a bathroom, and the medical stuff on the back wall for whatever. Someone did drag two chairs in, because one evening I had a roommate (less than 24 hours) who had pneumonia and her parents visited. Never mind I was still somewhat recovering from surgery, in immense pain, and possibly could be vulnerable to infections. Her parents were even wearing masks, as were the nurses and docs that came in when she was there. But there were no precautions for me, so I am thankful that didn't make it worse.

Within a few hours after being brought there, I was in a level of pain I had never been in before. I wanted to die. I had no control of my body when the back spasms hit. I would jerk and the spine would bend almost backwards. I couldn't sit up, much less stand, because I would just collapse. I had no lower body strength and everything below my ribs was painful beyond all belief. I pushed the nurse button several times, and honestly I am not sure how long it took for them to come in. The nurse came in with a little handheld device, checked it, said they were lowering my pain meds and I was going to have to deal with more pain than I had been at the other hospital. I noticed I had no catheter and I told her I needed to use the bathroom. She told me to grab the

IV fluid bag and go. I could not believe what I was hearing. I explained, through tears, that I could not sit up; I definitely could not stand up. She shrugged and said she would see what the doctor said and left. I waited, crying and hurting. I was already humiliated and scared out of my mind. I really did not want to pee the bed, though looking back, I probably should have and maybe they would have taken me more serious.

So I basically rolled off of the bed onto the floor, I cried and called out as I army crawled to the bathroom. I was almost at the door when a nurse came in and yelled for help. She was pissed at me for "acting out" and possibly hurting myself, in turn possibly getting her in trouble. They got me back into the bed and one of them came back with a sterile self-catheter and a plastic jug. She handed them to me and gave me something for the pain. I don't know what they gave me but it barely took the edge off. I used the self-catheter and peed in the jug. If you have ever done this, you know it is messy. You usually do it over a toilet or something because urine will come out around the catheter and the tube will have urine in it when you are done and that can spill too. It is messy. This is how I would have to use the bathroom for the next five days. The only thing I got was a new jug, if I happened to have filled mine up, and about once a day they would give me a new catheter. A lot of the stay is tinged shades of red. They would always have a reason why I could not have my pain medicine. At one point I was writhing on the bed, screaming as the agonizing spears of pain ripped up and down my back. A nurse came in, threw a wet rag at my face, told me to "clean up and stop being so damn pathetic", turned off the light and shut the door as she left. I saw one doctor that came in and said that he was a rheumatologist and I should make an appointment with him sometime about my fibromyalgia, and then he left. I tried to tell him what was going on and he said another doctor had my case. About twice a day I would get something in my IV that would help me sleep and take away a good portion of the pain, but often I would just get a lower level pain medicine that was not helping. I would pass out from exhaustion. I remember my face being on fire and raw from crying so much.

On the fifth day I was able to slide to the front of the bed and reach the phone. I called my spouse. He was sleeping in and didn't want to come up to the hospital. I told him I was scared and I wanted to come home. He got mad at me but said he would be up there shortly. He didn't show up until around lunch time, when I was brought my first tray of food. It was put on the table that can move over the bed, out of my reach, next to the three jugs of stale urine. When my spouse got there, the first thing he said was I looked awful and smelled really bad. We waited all day trying to get me discharged or transferred, and no one came in to see me. So I took out my IV and told my spouse to find a wheelchair. He did and we left. By the time he was getting me into the car, my cell phone rang. The hospital was pissed and wanted me to get back in there. I told them I removed the IV and left it on the table of pee jugs for them to inspect. I had some gauze held over it, and I was not going back in there ever again. When I got home I took some of my pain meds and found some relief but I couldn't walk without help or collapsing. And then I got the message that wonderful infectious disease doctor had left. She had been trying to call my cell phone for days and she knew what was wrong.

Looking back, I should have sued the hell out of that hospital. I should have had my spouse take pictures of my condition; I should have had him take me straight to another ER so I could be checked for infections or further damage or maybe just the state I was in after being in that bed dealing with what I had. I was dehydrated, hadn't ate in days, filthy beyond all belief, and very lucky not to have any infections. I learned about patient advocates after this. If I had known then, by law I could have requested one. If they refused me one, I could have called the cops on them. I did not know that. That knowledge helped me save my sister from a similar situation half a country away the next year. I will never forget that stay, though, and I never went back to that hospital. I was terrified and would get upset even thinking about it. I didn't sue because I didn't think I had proof. I was afraid they would say I was crazy and take me to an institution or something. I had to get the infection under control with the new doctor and I had a son to worry about. An institution was out of the question. But I could have done something. I could have called somewhere and gotten help. Do not let this happen to you. Demand a patient advocate. Everyone keeps cell phones on them, take pictures. If you have to, call the cops from your room. Do not let this type of abuse happen to you. It is illegal, wrong, and could be deadly and it will haunt you for the rest of your life if you get through it.

*A little bit about a doctor who almost killed me due to his inability to understand or speak decent English*: I feel that in this day and age of political correctness and everybody being offended by every damn thing that I need to make myself clear: I have nothing against foreign doctors/non-American doctors. In fact, the infectious disease specialist that saved my life and my awesome primary care doctor in Maryland were both from India and the amazing gastroenterologist who worked on my stomach, gallbladder and the Celiac Disease was African. That being said, I believe that in order to be a doctor who treats Americans, you MUST have a decent understanding of the English language. This story is a great example as to why.

This was back before everything went really bad, and back before I had my son. I was living in Florida with my former Spouse. I had really bad OCD, I mean, chasing people around the house sweeping up after them, barren and sparse furniture and things on shelves for easy cleaning; everything had its place and position, just really bad. My anxiety was also an issue. I would be fine one minute and the next minute my brain would start kicking out adrenaline and try to go into fight or flight mode for no reason. This causes a weird "split personality" effect. Part of you knows you are being illogical and that everything is fine and nothing is wrong. The other part of you thinks the world is ending, everyone hates you, everyone is doing something bad or dead, and it is just stupid ridiculous. Having a chemical based anxiety order is a mess. The excess adrenaline spins your brain into a strange place where it tries to come up with a reason why you need to go into fight or flight and starts making up scenarios like you are in a bad dream. Needless to say, I went to see a doctor.

I had not gone to a military approved doctor yet, much less seen any doctor in a while. So I made the appointment with the closest primary care manager to where we were living. When I got there, I waited forever and was finally called back by the nurse, nothing new, and sat in the examine room a while longer. When the doctor finally came in, it barely registered to me that he was Middle Eastern, I didn't really care. Then he started to talk to me. He had a very heavy accent and it was mixed by the wrong English words. I couldn't understand what this dude was saying! I told him a few times that I didn't understand and tried to relay to him what was wrong. He nodded a bunch and held up a finger and said something about medicine and being better. I nodded and told him that if medicine would help with the anxiety attacks I would try it. He went out and the nurse came back in with my prescription a bit later. I read the name and asked her what it was for. She told me depression. I asked her if that was treated the same as anxiety and she said yes. Well guess what, that is NOT true. Depression means too little adrenaline and anxiety is too much adrenaline, if you are given the medication of one for the other and it is something that focuses on adrenaline output, things can go bad, very bad.

I got the prescription filled and began taking it. On the third day I was starting to feel uncomfortable. I felt like my anxiety was getting worse and not better. I was worried the medicine wasn't working and called the doctor's office to make an emergency appointment to see if I needed to get off of that stuff before it messed me up. I went, I sat for five hours before I left in tears, angry and upset and having severe anxiety overload, and I had not seen the doctor. I went home and against my better judgement, took the medicine thinking it just hadn't had to take more time to work. Over the next few days, I remember my younger sister being at my house talking to me and another time my uncle banging on the door demanding I open up. Apparently I had messaged my spouse saying I wouldn't be there or anywhere when he came back from their training cruise. I had multiple anxiety attacks and was losing my damn mind. My sister and uncle stopped the medicine and within another few days I was feeling better again. I went back to the doctor's office and waited a long time again. Eventually I banged on the window and told the nurse I demanded to see my doctor. She asked what was wrong and I told her to be glad I hadn't killed myself due to the side effects of the medication he had given me. They told me to leave and I did. I got another doctor on base and saw her a few days later. The other doctor had wrote me down as severely depressed and low energy and had given me a medication known to cause suicidal tendencies and hysteria in anxiety patients. I should have sued him, or at least made him lose his license. He couldn't understand me and I couldn't understand him, thus I was misdiagnosed and given a medication that would have led to me doing something really stupid.

_A special kind of stupid: the nurse who wasn't a doctor_: I had a primary care "doctor" issued to me by the military when my former spouse was enlisted. We lived on base and so I saw her at the base hospital. This was after my pregnancy, before I moved to Maryland and found out my organs were falling out. Let me tell you, this woman was a joke! I do not remember much about her clearly, other than the fact she never told me she wasn't actually a doctor until I was trying to get medication later on and she couldn't prescribe it to me because only a doctor could prescribe it. I remind you, my organs were falling out! I saw this woman about once every two weeks for a month and a half until she infuriated me one day. Here is some of her diagnosis she gave me without even testing, blood work, examination, anything: ovarian cancer, uterine cancer, bad menstrual cycles, Leukemia, and whatever other cancer she could guess too. She would tell me she thought it was a random cancer, tell me we would need bloodwork and then say something completely different the next time. My last visit with her was almost comical. She huffed and sighed, tossing her blond hair around and rolling her eyes. She told me that her conclusion was that I was making a big deal out of a natural thing. She told me this: "All women have this ball of pain in their belly. I think you are focusing on the pain too much and letting it blossom to hurt you more than it should." I kid you not; I sat with my mouth hanging open, slid off the table, and shook my head as I walked out in complete disbelief. I went from her office straight to personal records department in the hospital and demanded my files. Later, when I went through them, I found out she had notes on each of my visits basically calling me an overweight hypochondriac. No medical diagnosis, no notes on her cancer statements to me (which would have me in a mess of fear and worry for a week) or any of that. Got to love those grade A idiots that are able to slip under the rope in the military.

_The doctor who would not be_: This one is super short, but a perfect example of how to deal with bullshit doctors. A little background to my situation, this was before the stomach issues in Georgia, but after my major abdominal surgery in Maryland. We were back in Florida for a few months, before we would lose everything and have to move. I had been diagnosed with Fibromyalgia, insomnia, migraines, anxiety, chronic nausea, chronic pain, etc. I was looking for a new doctor at the time. I had recently recovered from the massive surgery, the paralysis and infection, and all of that stuff. I knew my spine was badly damaged. I had dyed my hair for the first time in my life. It was black with a few dark blue stripes. I also had a new tattoo on my left forearm. My father had died a few weeks before from cancer. My parents were bikers and my mother was the tattoo artist. My sister was apprenticing for her and she was the one who had put my dad's memorial tattoo on my arm. I have to say, I knew nothing of the doctors in the area and picked this one off of my insurance list because her first name was Luna, and I thought that was kind of neat.

So I show up at the office in a t-shirt and jeans, my box of medical files and charts in my arms, my blue and black hair, and a newly healed tattoo. I checked in and sat in the waiting room. Shortly after the front desk clerk checks the chart, a pretty woman with long jet black hair, a skirt suit, and a doctor's coat walks out. She is holding files in her arms, the ones I had given the front desk at check in. She went to open the file and looked up as she called me name. Her hand froze when she looked at me, she closed the file, handed it to me and told me "I don't know why you came to see me, but whatever your problem is, I don't believe you." She then spun on her heel and walked back through the door she came in. I was stunned. I was crying by the time I got in the car and pissed beyond all belief by the time I got home. I called the county medical board, the main office at the clinic she worked for, and other medical boards and reported her to every single one for poor and unprofessional behavior and harassment. I am still stunned by how she acted, even years later.

# Living with Fibro

So now you know about dealing with doctors, the medicine available, what Fibro is and what it does. You know my story and you know a bit about dealing with the medical and legal issues. Now, how do you deal with it? How do you make it through tomorrow and tomorrow? Every day is different. Some days are decent, low pain and the fog is light and you feel like you can do something. If you have had Fibro for a few years, you are probably weary about pushing it. I have learned this and now I know better, though I still screw up from time to time. If possible, don't waste a good day busting your ass trying to get everything done. You will get this mind frame that you have to do all you can while you feel better because tomorrow might be bad. Let me tell you, my friend, if you do all you can today, tomorrow being bad is not a "might," it is a "for sure." Take each day as it comes. Most of what I know is because I have been dealing with this for a decade. I hate saying this, and I have had to say it to others before, a lot of knowing how to live with Fibromyalgia is time. Learning what you can do and what you can't. Learning who is there for you and who is not, how to respond to making plans, how to plan when you need to get something done, and so much more.

I am going to give some generic advice. Each one of us is different. We all have different family situations, partner situations, children, jobs, homes, hobbies, social groups, whatever, and so you have to tailor your needs to your life. I have a partner and live with him at his father's house. I do not have a job or car. My son lives with his father. I do not have much of a relationship with most of my family. My hobbies are sewing, crafting, reading, writing, playing video games, watching Netflix, cooking, making things, and that is about it. I do not have religious beliefs that include churches, so that is out. I do not have friends; I gave up on that long ago. I get on Facebook and I do have a Twitter because of the authors I review books for. I go to the store when the grocery situation is dire. I currently have a Tibetan Mastiff male dog we got from a rescue in Arizona named Oso, a Chihuahua/Australian Shepherd male puppy a friend asked us to take in named Krieg, and a fluffy part Maine Coon queen of the palace cat named Luna. And that is about it. So you have to adjust for how different your life and daily ins and outs are for you.

Here are some things that took time for me to learn, and my mother did always tell me the greatest lessons are lived and not told, so you will probably find out I am right the hard way, years from now.

First of all, people suck. I will explain more about this in the Support chapter under the "friends and family" heading. People will come and go. Do not ever feel guilty for this. It doesn't really matter, because if you are like me you will anyways, but it is not your fault. You did not decide to have this, there was no choice. Again, people suck. I eventually learned to tell people right off the bat that I had medical problems, I have a lot of bad days, and I can't do a lot so don't expect me to remember important days or events, actually show up if I say I might, or be dependable all the time. This usually clarifies things right away and can clear a room. As for dating, the first time I talked to my partner, I made it clear that I had scars, health issues, and was a mess. I felt that honesty warns them that I am not an easy person to deal with and cleared up any complaints later when I didn't live up to their manifested expectations.

Second of all, you can't do everything in one day and as I said before, you will regret it. I began trying to do everything I could when I was having a decent day or when I had good pain meds. As the symptoms racked up, the decent days lessened. I learned that if I did this, I would hate the next several days as I recovered. Your body does not function normally. That pain you feel is not the whole "muscle pain is weakness leaving the body" or some other bullshit. That pain you feel is because your body is confused and your wires are crossed and it is hurting whether something is wrong or not. Muscle pain with fibro doesn't mean a good work out, it means it hurts and you are making it worse, stop. Eventually, over time, I learned to micro manage. There are some good ideas on how to do this in the "Lifestyle Changes" section.

A big factor with Fibromyalgia is stress. Stress causes your muscles to tense up, your blood pumps faster, veins constrict, breathing is labored, and your stomach acids act up. These are just the physical reactions, but those reactions cause headaches, nausea, muscle cramps, dizziness, and other problems. There are also chemical reactions in your brain, such as higher adrenaline levels and lower dopamine levels. With Fibromyalgia, these are already an issue so those problems are amplified. I explain Fibro to people as if they didn't sleep for three or four days, got the flu and fell down the front stairs. What a person without Fibromyalgia deals with during stress will be ten times as bad as someone who does have Fibromyalgia. Lowering stress does in fact lower the pain. It also helps with sleeping and appetite levels. For me, I use marijuana for this. I used to be on Zoloft and Clonopin. Granted, I wish I still had the Clonopin for the nights where sleep will not happen. As I have mentioned before, I have gone up to four days unable to sleep. Even PM meds and Benadryl will not help when it is really bad. Stress makes this a definite possibility. I will discuss some lifestyle changes that could help with that in the following sections.

The big thing to remember is that many people may not understand what you are going through but that does NOT mean it is in your head or that it is any less severe than you feel it is. If it hurts, it hurts. If you are tired and can't think, you are tired and can't think so find a way to chill out. If you have young children, this can be a challenge, but there are ways to work with it. Your family needs to learn how to support you by doing the little things to make life easier. This may mean movie time so you can relax on the couch or an older child or spouse or family member watch them a day or more a week to help you have some time off to relax. Do not take on anything you do not think you can do. You may be proud and strong, but you have a condition that limits your body. Your body may feel like a concrete trap and I have said many times that I wish I could crawl out and away from it, if only for an hour. You can't help this; it is not your fault. If you need shortcuts, take them. If you need to sit around, do it. Who cares if someone says you are lazy? Tell them to jump off a cliff and then roll in drying cement and then get up and build a house. Then they can call you lazy.

## <u>Dealing with Skeptics, Nonbelievers, and those Hurtful Comments and Jokes</u>

"But you don't look sick."

"You just need a better diet and exercise."

"You were fine yesterday."

"Maybe you're just depressed."

"You're too young to have __________."

"My friend had that but she did __________ and is all better now."

"The doctor on __________ show says you just need __________."

"I think you're just too lazy/depressed/stressed."

"You look good today; I guess you're all better now?"

"Oh, you had __________procedure/surgery, so you should be fine now."

"Maybe you take too many medicines/pain pills."

"Aren't you afraid you will become a pill popper?"

"Shouldn't you try harder to do better?"

Ok, I can go on for pages with these stupid things people say. I have told you plenty of times and I will tell you many more, people suck. No one knows what you have been through, but you. No one has had the exact same circumstances, problems, medical history, or other aspects of your life. The most painful things will come from those closest to you. People you respect and love will cause the most hurt when they say things like this. Having any invisible illness is more difficult than those that have never had it could imagine. There are a few things you have to remember.

First, more than likely, the most they know is what they have read on social media or saw on some stupid television show. Don't get me started on the stupid doctor shows on television! They are not educational and feed on pop culture and trends, not science. Now, if they are the type of person not to listen to reason or read something you send them, then this won't really help. I would suggest looking up information on the Mayo websites or on legitimate college research pages and studies. Do NOT use Wikipedia to find information to build a legitimate case or teach someone about a disorder. This site, and all the sites related to it, are written, edited, and controlled by random people. WebMD is a little more authentic and supposedly uses people with some education or degree, but it is the internet and I don't trust that crap. You need to have facts, study results, and information that were created by people who have studied the issues. Real facts and real doctors are the source of legitimate information.

Second of all, how much about what you have been through does the person actually know about? If they are not close to you, not a friend or family member, screw them. You don't need that stress and explaining yourself to an idiot is a waste of time. If it is someone close to you, let them experience time with you when they normally won't. One of our downfalls, and yet biggest talents, is the fact that we wear masks. We can smile when we want to die. We can laugh when we want to cry. You need to let people in. I have had relatives that were not very concerned or interested in what I dealt with, but they wouldn't hesitate to make remarks behind my back about it. Give them a week of me staying with them or me calling when I am recovering from surgery or having a flare or fog day and making them come see me. You will be amazed at how quick their tune will change. I learned the hard way that faking it all the time is not good for you or the people around you. You will hurt yourself a lot and you will allow them to continue being assholes in their own ignorance. Let them know what it is like.

Tell them the bad stuff and how it really is. Let people in or they will never come close to understanding.

I just mentioned this briefly, but I think I need to make this completely clear, here: if the people that are giving you trouble are not close to you, get rid of them. Negativity will just hurt you. You cannot heal or lower your stress allowing people to be around who talk down to you, complain about you, or make comments or jokes at your expense. If your spouse has a friend that is a complete ass about your health, talks shit about you (even if he only does it when you are not present), then tell your spouse you do not want that person around you or your family. If it is a good friend or a family member of your spouse, then you need to sit down with your spouse and have a discussion. Does this person really know about your health and problems? If not, do they need to know? Can your spouse tell them that it is none of their business and that they would appreciate it if they didn't talk about what they didn't know? This is a very grown-up conversation, and as tough as it can be on you or on your spouse, this is you and your life. Rules need to be made and people need to understand, shut up or get lost. This applies to everyone you are in contact with. Make a decision based on whether they know the full story, whether they deserve or need to know, and if they can either not talk about something that is none of their business or they can get out of your life. It is harsh, but I can tell you that letting this happen only creates more pain and more torment later.

When it comes to the internet, do not get defensive. The whole idea of an internet "troll," someone who likes finding ways to pull people's strings or cause drama, is so ridiculous. Smart ass comments, rude memes or pictures, jokes, etc. should be ignored, removed or flagged, and the person needs to be blocked. I don't care if blocking them only means you won't see them. Who cares what they say? Who the hell are they? They are nobody. Do not give them bait or reason to provoke them. Be an adult and ignore, delete, and/or block. I know sometimes people will say things or do things on the internet that will just make you so damn mad. They will post fake "facts" or jokes or whatever because they think it's funny or they want to get a rise out of you. They want you to get mad, to get upset, and they want you to post your facts and excuses so they can prolong their fun little game. This is what they do. They have no life other than trying to make other people feel terrible so they can feel good about themselves. Let it go. I have fallen prey to this. I saw a stupid remark about people faking an allergy called Celiac towards gluten as an excuse, or some drivel like that. I had a bad day, wasn't feeling great, and I got mad. I started ranting about the pain I suffered and surgeries I needed and how much I missed Cheeze-it crackers and cheap pizza. It was pathetic and I eventually erased it when another troll jumped in and the two of them went off messing with me. It really is not worth it.

Professionals are the worst when it comes to this. Nurses, doctors, and pharmacists can be assholes too. Remember, you hire these people and you can fire these people. There are always more doctors and nurses and pharmacies out there. Finding a new one makes me nauseous just thinking about it, but I would rather do that then be ignored or badly treated by the very people who are being paid to help me. Although I do not like making a big deal out of things and taking it too far, you do have every right and can report them. The health department, your insurance, the hospital they work for, whomever. If someone is actually harassing you or refusing proper care, report them. If they are doing it to you then they are doing it to others and that is wrong. You can try to talk to them first, even warn them that you will report them if they do not act professionally, but if they fail to change, then go over their heads and make it clear that they are not doing well at their job. Harassment in medical facilities is a bad issue that many people won't talk about and too many people get away with. I have family in the medical field that has been asses to me about my condition. I have some that tell me stories about people they work with that are terrible with patients. I must say, though, just because a medical professional does not agree with you or is refusing to give you a medication you want, does not make them a bad doctor. If they do not have a legitimate reason for their behavior, then find another. This is not necessarily harassment or anything bad, just an inability to work together. Requests for medication that can do you more harm than good or your own refusal to listen to honest medical advice is not the professional's fault.

Remember that you have the right and the responsibility to either educate or eradicate. Help people understand you better or remove them from your life. Do not allow people to treat you badly. There is no reason to put up with it. I think the only person that has ever come to me that I had to help them deal with it was a young girl, mid-teens, who had Fibromyalgia and lived with a family member that was pretty nasty to her. All I could really do was try to help her see what other choices she had and help her learn how to block out the negativity. Limit people's access to you that do not deserve it. I will go further into dealing with family and close friends in the section under support. Remember: educate or eradicate!

## **Dealing with Fog**

Fibro Fog, oh how cottony and blurry you make me feel! Fibro fog is a nuisance more than anything, though it can cause problems if you work, attend school, or have mentally difficult things to do. The worst fog feels like a mixture between being drugged and having a stroke. There are days where I can't remember certain words or some sounds like ch might come out like sh. Reading or even trying to focus on what is happening on the tv can be difficult. You feel numb to most things. You can't focus, think, remember, or want to do any of those things. As someone who was once majoring in college on brains and their function, this can cripple you in some aspects. You basically go stupid. Function becomes minimal. What really pisses me off about

Fibro fog is that it doesn't mean you are necessarily hurting that bad, it just means that your brain is on the fritz.

So what should you do? Honestly, nothing. You can't, so don't. Lie around and watch tv, try to read, sit out and enjoy the day, or do something small and easy to do automatically. If you can nap, then nap. If you can push yourself to do some housework or some knitting or whatever, then do it. Don't drive if you do not have to. Don't go shopping if you do not have to. Try to minimalize any heavy thinking or concentration, because you don't need that stress. I know it is easier said than done, but you have to do this for you. You are not going to function well when you are in a Fibro Fog anyways, so do not try and force it. This will leave you more upset and possibly in more pain. Take it easy, you have a medical condition and sometimes you have to realize that it is something you cannot do anything about.

## Dealing with Pain

Fibro Flares can occur during a fog or on their own. Like a fog, they can last hours to weeks. Personally, my fog may last a day or two, but flares last anywhere from a day to a week for me. Stress, illness, surgery, and/or overdoing it can cause a flare. Sometimes, they happen for no reason. Flares are when the normal niggling pains and aches are amplified and really hurt or drive you to near insanity. If you have an old injury or another medical condition, it is possible for them to flare at the same time, or hurt more than normal. Sometimes a flare is not specifically a single bad pain, but maybe a multitude of uncomfortable issues. During my flares I may get that whole body sunburn feeling, where, as I mentioned before, it feels like you are covered in sand on top of the burn. It is irritating, and clothing, sheets, anything touching your skin just makes it worse. Sometimes a cool shower can help, but not always. A flare can also consist of all over bone, muscle, and/or joint pain. You may have a ridiculously long or painful headache. Basically, even if you feel like crap usually, a flare is when you feel like more crap than you usually would be feeling.

During a flare, pain medication can be wonderful. If you do not have access to pain medication or do not take medication, it can be difficult to deal with. Some people use yoga or meditation to help them. I have not found that this works for me. If it does for, that's awesome, do what helps you. Like a Fibro fog, you need to eliminate stress, or at least reduce it. I get moody when I am in a flare because it hurts, but also because I am frustrated with the nonsensical pain. I tell my partner as soon as I realize I am having a flare. This way he knows and he is expecting me to be aggravated, morose, upset, and probably immobile. Don't do anything you do not have to during a flare. This will only prolong it and make it worse. Once again, do NOT fault yourself or feel like you are lazy or anything like that. I must say again, it is a medical condition. It is not something you can control.

One of the ways I think about Fibro on a usual day versus a flare day is explaining how I deal with pain. If I really focused on how I feel on a normal day, I can pinpoint that my head is achy, my back hurts a bit, my muscles might be tender or sore, my feet could be bothering me, I might have itchy or irritated feeling, and so on. Over time, these little annoying things have kind of faded into background noise. It is like getting used to a bruise making a spot sensitive or a bug bite that you have finally stopped scratching at after hours of digging in your skin. It is the pebble you can't stop to take out of your shoe or a broken spring you always feel in your bed. It annoys you, it makes things difficult, but you have somewhat gotten used to it and now it is just a fly buzzing in your ear. In a flare, the straw breaks the camel's back. It is one push of pain, one more layer on the stack too much, and I am now feeling all of it. My head is pounding so much I can hear my blood pumping in my ears. My feet hurt so bad I keep looking at them thinking they are bleeding or black and blue. My back is so sore and achy I am afraid to bend to far or sit in the same position too long. Everything is cranked way up and the speakers feel like they are going to blow.

On flare days, you probably can't do anything even if you tried. With the fog, you may be able to push through a bit and get some stuff done. With a flare, you are better off finding a way to medicate, sleep, or maybe just hide in a cool dark room and beg for unconsciousness. I smoke marijuana, take Unisom PAIN or even Benadryl , try cool showers if I can handle standing that long (or warm or hot showers if I am more achy then burning/itchy), and lay curled up in bed. Trying to focus on a movie or tv show can help somewhat, pulling your focus away a bit. Sometimes, though, even that is not an option. Get someone to help you if you have young children or are alone. If you can't you may need to implement a "helper" day for your children. When you have a flare, they have to help you with things. When I taught early-preschool, I learned how useful this could be. Young children love to feel independent, special, and strong. Helping mommy is something they would happily do. Have them help you make sandwiches or make it a special "bowl of cereal dinner" day. One or two days not having a big cooked meal will not harm your child.

Just remember, "This too shall pass." The pain isn't going to be that bad forever. It will seem like forever, but it will go away. The sooner you can lower stress, relax, find a way to get some sleep, or any other way you can push through it, you will be back to your normal level again. My worst flares are on days following me pushing myself too hard: excessive walking, standing, big grocery trips, high levels of stress, when I am getting sick or already am sick, and then the wonderful random out of the blue moments. They will happen and they will suck and they will go away. I almost want to say "be strong," but honestly, anyone that has any kind of medical condition is a very strong person. What we deal with on a day to day basis, let alone what we deal with in flares, is enough to knock the strongest healthy adult on their ass. Our ability to deal with a hyper-sensitive nervous system does not make us weaker; on the contrary, it makes us much stronger simply because we have no choice. We have to get used to it or we will go insane and burn ourselves out. All you can do is what you are able to do without making anything worse. Coming from someone that has a terrible habit of putting others in front of me, you have to learn that you can't help or take care of anyone if you don't help and take care of yourself.

## <u>Personality Changes</u>

We would love to believe that who we are is not changed by our health issues. Believing that, though, will cause you more problems than it will solve. Despite my difficult childhood, I was still a very optimistic and easy going person. I am now very pessimistic and pretty much a loner. I savor my good moments. I may share them with those really close to me, but that is really it. I don't whine on social media or make a big deal out of procedures, surgeries, or even bad days. This is because of what I dealt with, though. There was a period of time, shortly after my diagnosis the first time and before I had the major surgery, where I would still call and talk to a lot of my family and I would post daily stuff on social media. Then people were always saying I was too negative and I was a downer. Well, you know what? I didn't have a lot of positive things to say. I was sick, I was hurting, I was changing and I was scared. I had to make some changes to that as well. So the biggest change is that your days will seem cloudier much more often then they will seem sunny and bright.

Your personality will also change because you will be changing. Things that didn't hurt before now hurt for seemingly no reason. You may not be able to do things that you used to do. Most of the time, regardless of how much you try, anxiety and/or depression will become part of your life. Anyone facing sudden changes to their daily plans, hobbies, abilities, and so on will not be pleased when those things are no longer an option. There are people out there that may not have gotten that severe. Perhaps you can still do your daily walk or your lifestyle is not greatly impacted. For you, I say bravo and I am genuinely happy that you are able to do so. Unfortunately, this is not true for the larger percent of people affected by Fibromyalgia. Plans are canceled, you go out less, and you don't feel comfortable doing all day events or trips because you know you could be exhausted and/or hurting afterwards. Sometimes even during events and trips. It is something you can't help but be unsure about. I would love to think I feel well enough to go get groceries and run errands and visit someone but I know that if I go alone, the driving will stress me because I get headaches and sometimes get confused when driving. Half way through the grocery trip I start hurting and begin to feel fatigued. Again if I am alone, my social anxiety kicks in and I begin to get stressed by the people around me.

The best thing you can do about feeling anxious or depressed is to find someone that you can talk to. You need a confidant, someone who will listen and not judge you. This is where online support groups have become an awesome source for me. I can talk to my partner, and I do. If I talked to him about every time I am anxious or depressed, though, I would become more stressed thinking I am burdening him with my sadness. I also know that he is there for me and he does not judge me, but he doesn't fully understand what I am going through personally. The people in my groups understand. They are there or they have been there. I have been a support just as much as people have supported me. I only talk about personal struggles and issues with my depression and anxiety in closed groups. These groups are not visible to other people. My mom or even my partner's mom, even my partner unless I show him, can't see what we talk about or what is posted in those groups. We can talk about suicide, depression, abuse, and any other dark topic. We also talk about good things and events, ask questions about symptoms and medication, find out information about surgeries and procedures, ask about issues with going to the bathroom or sex, anything we want to ask about. They even have a neat international secret Santa thing every year. I would suggest looking for one, if you can and if you have regular internet access. Some areas have local groups, but these are few and far between. Mostly because people with Fibromyalgia are not often able to go to a weekly meeting, or do not want the face to face contact. Once again, I will go more into friends that you can talk to under the support section.

Whatever you do, remember that change happens. It really doesn't take a whole lot to change a person's behavior and personality, and something as major as a lifelong condition of pain and exhaustion is going to be reflected in who you are. We can wear our masks, we can put on the plastic smiles, but underneath we are still hurting. My son and my partner are the only two people who can see past my mask. Both of them will call me out when I say I am okay because they tell me they can see the pain in my eyes. The most difficult part of my change is that it did have an impact on my relationship with my ex-husband. This, very unfortunately, is more common than any of us like to see. I see it in my groups, I get private messages about it, and I see it posted on pages of other Fibromites. Relationships break or become stronger, there is no real in between if you want to not live a very stressful existence. I like to believe that my health issues are almost a truth serum for people. I quickly can find out who a person really is by how they deal with me, especially at my worse.

## <u>Lifestyle changes</u>

Lifestyle changes are like the personality changes, they will happen. I recently read an interesting article in which a woman was actually thanking her Fibromyalgia for teaching her how to reduce stress, get rid of people who were not worth the pain, and for changing how she looked at the world. At first I thought the article was a bit silly, but as I read through, I understood what she meant. Once you know that you have Fibromyalgia, and the knowledge of why you are always tired and hurting makes since, you can find comfort that it is not something you are doing wrong or being lazy about. Then, you have to get that through your head: you are NOT lazy or weak! Now you have to go through any mourning and acceptance that your life is changing and that you will have to make more changes. When that is out of your system, it is time to make those changes and stick with them.

You can't do as much, you have days where you can't do anything, and over time, the simplest task will be more difficult. The best way to deal with changes to your lifestyle is to make them happen on your own time. Don't force yourself to work until you drop dead or go to every event you are invited to until you are physically unable to attend. Instead, think about where you are at, what you can do without pushing yourself to hard, and cut back to that mark. Answer "maybe" on invitations, so that you do not feel as bad if that day is a flare or fog or some other reason prevents you. I am not saying quit doing things or going places or leave your weekly book club, I mean stop setting your expectations too high so you end up crushed when you find you cannot do it. You may not have a choice about having Fibromyalgia, and you may not have a choice in how it limits you, but you do have a choice in how much those limitations impact you.

<u>Meal Time</u>:

Make dinners on days you feel well and freeze them for fog and flare days. Or make your rough days a pizza day. Plan ahead to have meals for your kids prepped for days when your function will be at its lowest. The same goes for you. Have meals you can easily heat up. Planning ahead is a wonderful way to help you through these bad times and is a lot easier than you probably give it credit for. My partner keeps frozen pizzas and meals in the freezer (I can't have the gluten filled frozen stuff) to cook and eat on days I am having a fog or flare. Usually I am not feeling up to eating at all so I might have some fruit or something. Crock pot meals or something you can put in the oven together (like a roast with vegetables) makes not only a decent large meal, but is something easy to partition out and even freeze. When I cook, I try to make double what we will eat so I can freeze half of it. Then on rough days, I can pull out the frozen meal and heat it up in the microwave, oven, or in a large pot on the stove at a low heating level.

Use timers on the microwave or the little electronic ones that go off when the food needs to be checked or turned off. Some of the newer kitchen appliances even have settings that make it turn off on its own after a certain time. You can even set a timer or alarm on your phone or computer or set an actual bedside alarm next to you. There is a good possibility, especially on a bad day that you might forget that you are cooking. Use the wonderful technological devices we have to help you, which is why we have them.

Cleaning:

There are several little shortcuts and things you can do to make cleaning a simpler task. You do not need to clean the entire house in one day. Make Mondays the bathroom day and Wednesday is vacuuming, or whatever works for you. For me, the bathroom usually needs to be thoroughly cleaned once every two weeks (if you have children or messy boys, try to get them to clean up their own mess). So I keep the toilet brush by the toilet and run it around the inside of the bowl every few days. I sweep the floor once every seven to ten days unless it really needs it. I scrub the tub using a very unsafe method of a blue toilet cleanser in a squirt bottle (do not breathe that in or get it on your skin) and a sponge mop on a handle. I wipe the counters down every few days. Clothes can, in fact, sit in a basket for a few days, and this killed me for a while because I used to have severe OCD and had to put them away immediately. Needless to say, I got over my OCD really fast after a baby and then Fibro. Find shortcuts. If you are poor like me, make short cuts. For instance, you can buy Clorox wipes or make your own. Ripped up rags or old socks can be kept in an old butter container or wipes container with a vinegar and water solution to clean with like wipes. Use a Swiffer for floors (I use a generic brand that you can fill the reusable container with hot water or cleanser or whatever). Sponges make great dishwashing utensils because as long as you rinse them, if they are not falling apart, zapping them in the microwave for five minutes will kill off the bacteria and keep them from getting icky and stinky. Keep cleansers in the room you use them in inside of a basket or in a cabinet or something. This makes it easy to spot clean and you don't have to carry so much back and forth. Simplify, there is absolutely no reason not to, even if you were perfectly healthy!

<u>Children</u>:

Taking care of your children when you have Fibromyalgia is exhausting. If anything, I think this is one of the greatest challenges. One of the hardest things to overcome is your pride. There is nothing wrong with asking for help. Albeit family, your spouse, older children, or whomever you can get to help you, just ask. You are not relinquishing your ability to take care of them or being less of a parent if you ask someone to watch them while you take a nap or on a really bad day where the pain or fog is too much. For a while, when I was recovering from surgeries and having a hard time in an old, dilapidated home on the mountain, I had my brother's teenage step-daughter staying with me. I was home schooling her and helping her with her advanced classes and she would help me with my son and with doing things around the house. That is on the more extreme end, as I was doing something in return and there were other circumstances to why we were doing things that way. This does show you that you do not have to fear the need of other people helping, as many others need help too.

Logically, though, you will not always have someone to help. Like with meals, and as I mentioned earlier in the book, plan ahead. Have a basket or drawer of activities for elementary aged children (books, coloring stuff, board games, those little science kits, etc.) that they can do with just simple supervision. With younger children, you have to watch them constantly and you have to do everything for them when they are babies or toddlers. This is when child gates, child-proof door locks, and having child safe areas in your home are great. As long as you have a comfortable place to sit with them, and they have what they need, there really isn't too much you have to worry about. My biggest scare, and something that happened to a woman I used to know, was that she fell asleep while her toddler had run of the house. She had no child locks or a safe area for the child to play in, and he went right out the front door and the military police on the base were called. Just because you may be sleepy or your medicine makes you sleepy, does not give an excuse to be unsafe. If anything, have a chain lock, or even a deadbolt, installed at the top of your doors. If the play room or area has its own separate door, you can use an inexpensive hatch and just stick a lock through it, there is no need to actually lock it (a lock is just safer than a screwdriver that can be knocked out), so that they can't go wandering around the house if you fall sleep in there with them.

Smart thinking, awareness of your child, and preparation beforehand will make taking care of children easier when you are not feeling well. Rarely are you going to be sick or in a fog for more than a few days, even that long. Usually you may have a day or two where you will need precautions like this, and hopefully you do have people that can help you. If you don't, though, there is no reason for you to be worried or feel bad for making things easier for you and safer for your child. Honestly, I do not think it is terrible to lock yourself in the play room with your little one if you are tired. As long as the room is safe, and you are not medicated to where you will be sleeping hard (any mother I know usually only light naps around their young, you are kind of programmed to react to them instantly). I do not condone leaving young children alone or unsupervised. I also do not agree with taking medication that will make you drowsy or sleepy when you have young children around. Not being able to take stronger pain medication is hard, but if you have a young child, their wellbeing may mean you have to tough it out for a few hours.

<u>Being Out of the House</u>:

This may seem like an obvious thing to say but if you are not feeling well, you are in pain, your fatigue is high, or you feel stressed out, do not leave home unless it is an emergency or very important. It bugs me that I may want to go to the grocery store today but I am too tired or sore. I get really aggravated when it is two days later and I still do not feel like going. So on days that I am feeling good, I make a decision between cleaning, or doing errands. When I am feeling like I am at my best condition to go deal with people and the grocery store, I go. I am so happy for 24 hour super centers because sometimes it is 3am when I make this decision. If you can get someone to go with you, then bring them along. You can ask your spouse, older child, friend, or family member to ride along with them or for them to go with you if you need support. If you do not have issues with anxiety or health issues that can be bad when you are alone, then don't worry about having people with you. That is a preference thing and for me it has to deal with my bad social anxiety and my issues driving.

Limit the number of places you need to go. Try to make the least amount of stops that you can. That being said, I suggest the most difficult and necessary stops first. If I need to go to the grocery store and I need to get new shoes soon, I will do the grocery store first. It is going to take the longest, cause the most amount of stress, is the more necessary trip, and if I am exhausted afterwards, I can just go home and worry about shoes another day. Plan smart. I try to make one big grocery trip every two to three weeks. On that one, I have my partner come with me and we go to a super center and get the bulk packages of toilet paper and cleaning supplies, pet food, and large amounts of freezer stuff, dry and canned food, and then a decent amount of the perishables. I do not like having to go to the grocery store every day or every other day just to make a meal or pick up something I forgot. I make a massive list and try to get as much as I can in a big trip. I have a dry erase board on the fridge to write down anything I need or we run out of so I can plan to get that on the trip. Keep a notebook in the kitchen if you don't have a dry erase board or one of those magnetic lists on the fridge.

If you begin to not feel well, start hurting, or are getting tired, it is time to wrap it up: finish getting what you really need, check out, and go home. Once again, there is no need to push yourself until you break. Do not go to places or to events where you are going to stand or walk a lot unless you know there will be places to sit and rest, or you really know that you can do it without hurting yourself. Stubbornness will not make the pain easier or the fatigue less, you will just hurt yourself.

My point, in this book, is not to discourage you or tell you that you can't do something, but to remind you that when you are limited, if you are limited, that there is nothing to blame but biology, nature, and genetics. If you do not need to make short cuts yet, if you are still able to push through a lot, then do so. Never feel bad, though, if you can't. Don't get mad with yourself when you do have to start setting limits. Everyone, eventually, needs limits. We are just unfortunate enough to have to set those limitations earlier than some people. Just remember, you can prevent problems by preparing yourself, your home, and your family to make things easier for all of you. Make the shortcuts a part of life; slowly implement them into everyday living so that it isn't such a big change. As I mentioned before, even if you didn't have Fibromyalgia, it never hurts to make things easier for yourself.

## <u>Coping Mechanisms</u>

Now you are making changes, you have systems in place for the bad days and you are doing what you can when you can. You understand that sometimes the day is not going to go as you were planning for it to go. Fogs and flares are days that pop up whenever they want and you are getting more comfortable with the idea that you can relax and take it easy when this happens. Regardless of all of these things, there will be moments where it is just so overwhelming. The limitations, the changes, the inabilities to do what you want when you want can catch up to you. So what do you do? How do you deal with crushing anxiety or depression or both? What can you do when it all seems like too much?

I can't say this enough, but it is not your fault. You don't want this, you never would have asked for this, and none of it is your choice. It may sound redundant, you may think I have said this way too many times, but I still get sucked into my own head and find myself apologizing for a medical disorder. I know it's not my fault and I know I can't help it but I feel guilt when it affects other people. I hate that, I feel like a burden. My partner tells me constantly not to apologize for it, and that it isn't my fault. It's just one of those things that you have to pound into your head until it becomes a solid imprint in your mind.

Secondly, if it is someone else that is making you feel depressed or anxious about your health or how you are dealing with it, you need to do something about that. Talking is always the first route. Keep an open line of communication. You should be able to confidently tell your partner or close family members that you are having a bad day or you are in a flare or fog and they know what it means. No questions, no second guessing you, they understand. If they don't, then perhaps they are closer than they need to be. I have cut out entire sections of my family because of this. I have dropped almost all of my "real life" friends. Negative people, mean people, assholes, miserable people that want you to join in their misery are not worth the pain. It hurts and it can be rough to tell someone you do not need them around, but it is worth it in the long run. If a person really cares about you, they will understand and either try to help you or leave you alone. Someone nagging you or blaming you for things, they are not looking to help they are only going to hurt. I have mourned the loss of friends and family after I have cut them out, but once I got over their absence, it was a breath of fresh air not to have the constant nagging, blaming, accusations, cruel words, and whatever else they wanted to throw at me. I would rather be alone and grow stronger in my will and my own understanding than be surrounded by people that either never help or only help by making me miserable. No thank you.

So removing people and self-blame from the equation, what if you do find yourself still overly distraught, upset, anxious, depressed, bawling and you don't know why? This is where we get into actual coping mechanisms. Many people will say that you should meditate or relax. Oh my, the laughter that bubbles up with that one. I am all about meditation and relaxation techniques, but I can't do it. I have insomnia, and I will lay there in the dark for hours trying to think happy thoughts or try not to think of anything. This doesn't work for me. I have researched Zen and mindfulness. This stuff isn't for everyone. I have to say, though, a lot of Buddhist, Confucius, Shinto, and Zen techniques can be very handy.

Mindfulness is one of the most effective methods I have found. The basic idea is to quite your mind by filling it up. You focus on any and everything around you that doesn't hurt. The way the sheet feels on your legs, the breeze on your face, and the cool and sweet flavor of your drink, the shadows and lines the light makes on the walls, and so on. You focus on all these little details. I used to have a bad habit of staring off into space and my mind would swirl down the dark drain into thoughts that would upset me or sadden me and I would just keep sinking. Now, when I catch myself doing that or find I am overwhelmed by thoughts, I start focusing on every sensation. One really easy way to force a lot of feelings and sensory events is to eat or drink something complex. If you are able to have wine or a rich and natural ice cream or cheese, something that has certain textures and layers of flavor you can really let yourself sink into them. Chocolate is amazing if you like getting different flavors and types of chocolate bars. I like rich dark red wines, rich heavy cheddar cheeses, dark chocolate, savory meats, and fresh fruit. Cool pools, relaxing scented baths, soft lotions that have a light fragrance; things like this are great to focus your senses on. I put lotion on twenty times a day, a soft floral St. Ives. It is smooth, dries quickly, smells good, and gives me a few minutes of sensory distraction. Whatever works for you, whatever makes your mind focus elsewhere. After about a week of doing this, I noticed an obvious difference in my state of mind. I was less stressed and didn't get depressed as often because I didn't give myself time to sink into that darkness.

Then there are those times where you are a mess. Not a sad feeling or thinking too much, just a full blown blast of tears and heartache that you can't stop. During these breakdowns there are three ways to deal with it. If you are on medication for it (including Clonopin, Valium, or even marijuana) take what you are prescribed or your usual dose and let it set in. Second option is to cry it out, in a cool shower if you can, and then sleep it off. Third option is to have a reliable person you can have in person, on the phone, through text, on a support group, or however you communicate with them. Make sure they know ahead of time that during these situations you need distraction and comfort. If anything, have a code word. My partner knows when I am going through one and immediately takes action. If it is an angry cry, he stands back, lets me rant, and then comforts me when I run out of steam. If it is a depressed, distraught cry, he immediately comforts me and then distracts me with conversation. Sometimes it is silly stuff, sometimes deep thought provoking conversations, sometimes it is about a movie or book or game. The key here is to know what you need and to have someone who knows this and can help you through it. If you don't have someone you can trust at home, seriously check out the Fibromyalgia forums. Post a message asking for help or for someone to talk to. Tell them that you don't need "it will be ok" or any of that. Tell them what you need and someone will come forward and help you. In one of my secret groups, there is always someone up and on Facebook. If one of us posts we are having a rough time and need someone, there is eight people there for him or her. I have ten friends on my friend list that are just fibro friends that we message each other when things are bad or when we have questions or anything like that.

If you are experiencing a lot of anxiety and/or depression, you do need to adjust things in your life to make an overall less stressful situation. Fibromyalgia makes schedules hard, so trying to make a specific bed time or relaxing time is usually impossible. If you like herbal teas and they do not clash with your medicine (and you have no allergies to them) try chamomile teas. You can add lavender, mint, orange, cinnamon, honey, or whatever you like. Warm tea is very relaxing. Another relaxing drink is honey and milk heated up in the microwave. Make sure you do it in 15 second bursts so you do not scald the milk. I have also added dehydrated peanut butter powder to it as well and it worked nicely. Aromatherapy candles, oils and incense are also nice. Scent can have a huge effect on atmosphere. Pick comforting scents or relaxing scents. You can also buy or make an eye pillow. I use a silky material and flax seeds. I cut the material to about 7 inches by 10 inches. I fold it in half, inside out, to make it 3.5 inches by 10 inches. I sew up one side and the bottom side and then half of the last side. I turn it right-side out, fill about ¾ of the way full with flax seed (you can also toss lavender buds in with this) and sew up the last part. You can lay back and put this over your eyes and it is amazing. It is the perfect weight for headaches too. Silky materials will always feel cooler, as well, making it even more comfortable. I may be writing a book soon on comfort and relaxation techniques, especially for people dealing with anxiety and depression.

Depending on how bad your depression and anxiety is, you may need to talk to your doctor. In severe situations medication may be better for you. I am not crazy about medication, but most of my anxiety is more chemical and hormonal then mental. So medication is necessary to keep those chemicals and hormones in balance. Again, it isn't for everyone, but I do find that marijuana can help with this a lot. If you have anxiety issues and can easily panic, do not try any cannabis products alone and start in small doses. There is a possibility, for some people that marijuana will actually increase or kick off anxiety attacks due to the ability for it to cause paranoia. Also, learn about cannabinoids. There are different strains for different things. *Indicas* have a higher *CBD* level and a lower *THC* level and are better for medical use. They do not cause much of a psychoactive effect and are used for depression, nausea, migraines, headaches, pain, and muscle spasms. *Sativa* has a higher THC level and a lower CBD level and causes a more psychoactive high. Sativa is considered almost an artistic high as people can be more active, more imaginative, stimulated, thoughtful, and focused when using it. In the defense of this controversial plant, it is a hell of a lot safer than the majority of any medications we often find ourselves taking. It doesn't cause liver damage or heart failure, extremely difficult and almost impossible to ever overdose on, and is milder and not as strong on the body as pharmaceuticals. Regardless of whether you like CBD oil or smoking a joint or taking a Valium, if it helps you regulate depression and anxiety, use it. That is why these things are available to us.

## Family and Friends

I felt it necessary to make a separate topic about dealing with family and friends. They can either be our biggest and best support network, or the main reason for our depression and anxiety. I have gone over how important it is to weigh the good versus the bad and that sometimes it is necessary to cut the bad from your life. Now I want to focus on the good and how you can properly balance needing family and friends and not coming off as overly needy. Over time, needing someone to support you is something you will have experience with. Sometimes, you will find a friend or you will be lucky and have an amazing family and they will always be there for you, never question you or look down on you, and will hold you up when you are falling down. Unfortunately, this can take its toll on people. Yes, it's true that we may not have good news to share or good things to talk about, we may be rather negative. On many occasions, I discovered I didn't call my mom or some other family member very often only because I felt I was always too negative or all I had to talk about was my health problems. When it was brought to my attention that I rarely called and when I did I had nothing but complaints and bad news, I realized I was just making it worse.

It took me a lot longer than it should have to figure out that what I needed to do was force myself to call for no reason at least once in a while, and just talk. I made it a point to ask how they were and what they had been doing. I was short on answers about my situation or I would make a big deal out of something positive like a special dinner I made. A ten to twenty minute phone call that only focuses on the supporting person can do a lot for that person. It makes them feel appreciated and lets them know you do care about them. With all that we go through, the crazy in our minds and our bodies, it is hard to slow down and look around us at the people who are there, but it is important that we do. Randomly make or buy some cards telling them how much you appreciate them being there for you and how important that is to you. Do not go off and start writing "because I am always sick" or "since I have this problem and this problem" or anything similar. Try to leave all of your problems out of these showings of appreciation. Random positive calls, small cards or gifts as a thank you, and kind words to those that are there for you are what will make sure they are happily there for you in the future.

## Facebook Groups

- Young People Living with Fibromyalgia/Chronic Pain - https://www.facebook.com/groups/123134957844771/

- Fibromyalgia/CFS Fighters Group - https://www.facebook.com/groups/188638827882074/?ref=browser

- Chronic Pain - https://www.facebook.com/groups/ChronicPain.MyLife/

## Websites and Organizations

- The Fine Print of Pain – http://thefineprintofpain.wordpress.com[1]

- American Pain Foundation - http://www.painfoundation.org/

- National Fibromyalgia & Chronic Pain Association - http://www.fmcpaware.org/

- Social Security Disability - https://www.ssa.gov/disabilityssi/

- Patients Like Me - https://www.patientslikeme.com/

## Books

- How to be Sick by Toni Bernhard

---

1. http://thefineprintofpain.wordpress.com/

Mayo Clinic – https://www.mayoclinic.org[1]

Medical Dictionary – https://medical-dictionary.thefreedictionary.com[2]

1. https://www.mayoclinic.org/

2. https://medical-dictionary.thefreedictionary.com/

# Don't miss out!

Visit the website below and you can sign up to receive emails whenever Amanda Leanne publishes a new book. There's no charge and no obligation.

https://books2read.com/r/B-A-ERBF-FWNP

BOOKS2READ

Connecting independent readers to independent writers.

# Also by Amanda Leanne

Shadows Through the Fog
The Fine Print of Fibro
Sever the Circle
Mind the Mirrors

Watch for more at https://amandaleanne.com/.

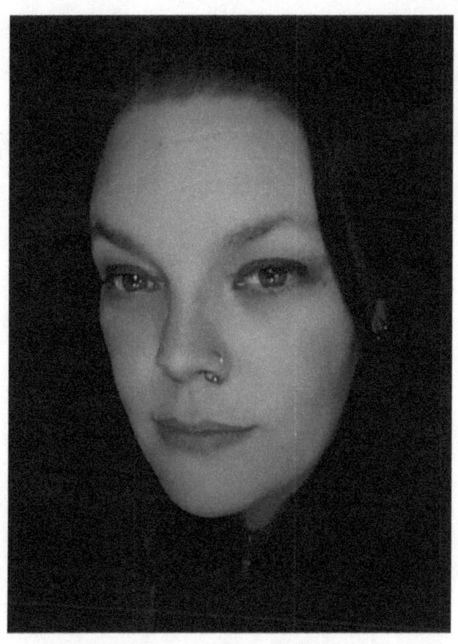

# About the Author

Amanda Leanne began reading at a very young age and has been writing since grade school. She is a prolific reader, book collector, and writer with an interest in all aspects of art including sewing, painting, sculpting, jewelry design, soapmaking, and various other hobbies. After spending nearly a decade working on her degrees in forensic sciences, abnormal behavioral science, and neurological psychology with the prospect of joining the FBI ViCAP unit, Amanda's health took a turn for the worse. Daily struggles with her medical issues hasn't stopped her from pursuing her childhood aspirations to become an author. She currently lives with her spouse (Kris), her son, and their cats in the mountains of Northern Alabama. Leanne writes non-fiction as well as fictional novels. Her non-fiction books and articles delve into topics such as medical conditions, true crime, psychology, and crafting. Her fictional stories delve into horror, psychological, mystery, thrillers, eerie tales, science fiction, and paranormal worlds.

Read more at https://amandaleanne.com/.